£ 3 —
MM
19/45

Changing Patterns of
Conception and Fertility

Changing Patterns of Conception and Fertility

*Proceedings of the Sixteenth Annual
Symposium of the Eugenics Society
London 1979*

Edited by

D. F. ROBERTS
*Department of Human Genetics,
University of Newcastle upon Tyne, England*

R. CHESTER
*Department of Social Administration,
The University, Hull, England*

1981

Academic Press
A Subsidiary of Harcourt Brace Jovanovich, Publishers
London · New York · Toronto · Sydney · San Francisco

ACADEMIC PRESS INC. (LONDON) LTD.
24/28 Oval Road,
London NW1

United States Edition published by
ACADEMIC PRESS INC.
111 Fifth Avenue
New York, New York 10003

British Library Cataloguing in Publication Data
Changing patterns of conception and fertility.
1. Fertility, Human — Congresses
I. Roberts, D.F. II. Chester, R.
304.6'3   HB903.F4

ISBN 0-12-589640-9

LCCCN 81-66700

Text set in Singapore by Colset Private Limited
and printed in Great Britain by T.J. Press (Padstow) Ltd

Contributors

R. J. BEARD, *Consultant Gynaecologist, Royal Sussex County Hospital, Brighton, England*

BERNARD BENJAMIN, *Department of Mathematics, The City University, London, England*

M. A. FERGUSON-SMITH, *Department of Medical Genetics, University of Glasgow, Scotland*

D. F. HAWKINS, *Institute of Obstetrics and Gynaecology, Hammersmith Hospital, London, England*

H. S. JACOBS, *Department of Obstetrics and Gynaecology, St Mary's Hospital Medical School, London, England*

PETER LASLETT, *Cambridge Group for the History of Population and Social Structure, Cambridge, England*

M. C. MACNAUGHTON, *Department of Obstetrics and Gynaecology, University of Glasgow, Scotland*

J. R. NEWTON, *Queen Elizabeth Medical Centre, Birmingham, England*

JOHN PEEL, *Teesside Polytechnic, Middlesborough, England*

J. K. RUSSELL, *Department of Obstetrics and Gynaecology, University of Newcastle upon Tyne, England*

SUE TEPER, *Department of Community Medicine, University of Nottingham, England*

B. VIEL, *International Planned Parenthood Federation, London, England*

Preface

This volume contains the thoroughly edited texts of papers presented at the Sixteenth Annual Symposium of the Eugenics Society held in September 1979. The second in a trilogy examining changing patterns of biological variables in contemporary society, this volume is devoted to the fundamental biological processes of conception and fertility. From it, a collection of statements by authorities studying these processes from widely different points of view, fertility can be seen for what it is: an objective of all-pervasive concern. At the individual level there are the problems engendered by fertility which is too prolific, the worries of fertility which is absent, too low, too early, or too late, and the difficulties of looking after the less healthy products of that fertility. Similar problems arise, on a different scale, at the community and the world level. It becomes evident from each individual paper how the great changes that have occurred in fertility have brought many new and unexpected problems, both biological and social. The volume is far from comprehensive but it gives the thinking reader some indication of the variety of problems involved and many points to ponder, while those professionally engaged in family medicine will find the definitive discussions in the latter half valuable reference reviews.

The symposium examined four main topics. Fertility in its demographic context is first examined, Professor Benjamin drawing attention to the merits and demerits of the different measures of fertility, the secular changes that have occurred in fertility in Britain, and the factors influencing them. Professor Viel discusses the quite different situation in the contrasting historical background of Latin America, with particular reference to political motivations, and shows clearly the vicious net of high fertility, poverty and ignorance into which so much of the population has become enmeshed. Here also comes the text of the Society's Galton Lecture of 1979, given by Mr Peter Laslett, viewing through an historian's eye the apparently inexorable demographic march of man. The questions he poses in it are justification enough, if justification were needed, for the theme of the symposium as a whole.

The second part is devoted to the prevention of fertility, and so represented both achievement and assessment of its results. Dr Peel reviews the development of family planning and attitudes to it over the last century, and shows that the most usual methods of the present are, with the exception of the use of oral contraceptives, those of the past. Dr Jacobs looks into the foreseeable future, and argues that those of the future will essentially remain those of the present, despite several exciting developments. The definitive paper by Sue Teper, besides containing much material published for the first time, gives an objective assessment of the risks of the several contraceptive methods, so that information, guidance and support can be given to individuals when making their choice.

With the potential, already almost fully realized in many Western countries, for couples to control the number of their children, it is appropriate that they be able to improve the quality of their fertility. Professor Macnaughton discusses recent advances in the causes and treatment of involuntary childlessness; particularly distressing psychologically and socially to those couples who suffer from it. Professor Ferguson-Smith examines the present possibilities for avoiding serious birth defects and shows how prenatal diagnosis early in pregnancy, followed by termination where the foetus is shown to be affected, can appreciably reduce the birth incidence of several types of defect. Mr Hawkins is concerned with one group of controllable insults to the developing foetus and infant, and he gives an authoritative summary of the effects of drugs in pregnancy and lactation; his wise words both of reassurance and caution will be useful particularly to those who are responsible for prescribing.

The final section is devoted to areas of current concern for the unexpected problems to which they are giving rise. Professor Newton draws attention to the extent of artificial insemination by donor, examines the complex legal issues and reviews the research that has been carried out into methods and success; he shows how little is really known, and the need for much more comprehensive clinical research into AID. Professor Russell discusses the distressing recent rise in the number of pregnancies among young schoolgirls, and examines some of the immediate long-term problems faced both by them and their families. Finally, Mr Beard examines the risks and problems to the older parent, particularly the mothers, not only in the pregnancy but also during and after delivery and in the subsequent development of the child; he ends on an optimistic note, that with good care and perhaps with greater supervision, one can expect a favourable outcome and the older woman need not be deterred from having a pregnancy.

Altogether there were over 250 participants in the symposium, and the informal discussions that took place during the two days made clear that its first object, of stimulating thought and provoking discussion among those present, was indeed achieved. It is hoped that this volume will do the same among those who were not fortunate enough to be present.

The editors acknowledge with thanks the great help given by Miss Eileen Walters in the organization of this symposium, and the preparation of this volume.

on behalf of the Eugenics Society
D. F. ROBERTS
R. CHESTER

MARCH 1981

Contents

Recent and Prospective Fertility Trends in Great Britain

BERNARD BENJAMIN

Department of Mathematics, The City University, London, England

Because more detailed statistics over a longer time are available for England and Wales, this chapter refers often to that part of Great Britain. It is of course the major part, accounting for 90 per cent of the total population. Thus though the general level of fertility is somewhat higher in Scotland than in England and Wales, this is not enough to produce a significant difference between measures for the latter country and those for Great Britain as a whole.

Concepts and Definitions

When we speak of fertility we refer to the births delivered of a woman during her reproductive life-time; to the extent to which her ability to bear children (her fecundity) is actually exercised. A woman can now choose*, with increasing but not total effectiveness, whether she will bear children at all and, if she does decide to bear children, the points of time during her reproductive life at which these births shall occur. The births which actually occur in this country in any one calendar year are those parts of the total fertility of women born in different years (members of different generations) and married in different years (members of different marriage cohorts) which they allocate by design (or accident) to that year without telling the Registrar General (even if they knew) what fractions of their eventual complete families those parts might be. So the total births in the year and, therefore, the official birth-rate (which is simply the ratio of that number of births to the total population), though useful in conjunction with the death-rate as a measure of the rate of population growth in the year, is not a measure of

---

* For the purpose of this discussion which is concerned only with statistical measures of fertility, I am ignoring the male partner's part in this decisionmaking.

the fertility level. It does not relate to a specific generation or marriage cohort and it is liable (increasingly so as freedom of choice, for a woman, increases) to be strongly influenced by changes in the timing and pace within marriage of the family building process. If the average family size remains constant but women decide to start their family building earlier and complete it more quickly, then births that would have occurred later are brought forward in time and the birth rate rises, as it did in 1955. Such a rise in the birth-rate persists only until the new timing has established itself for the average number of years (about ten) over which families are thereafter built and the birth-rate (other things being equal) begins to revert to its former level, as it did in 1965. Again if the average family size remains constant but women decide to postpone the start of family building or to postpone later (i.e. higher order) births, then we have the reverse of the 1955 change in timing and the birth-rate falls. There is reason to believe that this kind of change in timing added to the decline in the birth-rate after 1965. The same kind of change in timing is imposed by the wartime separation of husbands and wives and the deterrent to family building of war conditions, as after 1914 and after 1939. When war ends these births are rapidly made up and there is a sharp peak in the birth-rate as in 1920 and 1947. These increases and decreases in the birth-rate as a result of changes in the age of onset and in the subsequent pace of family building may be sharpened or blunted by other changes. For example if the norm of family size is not constant but is declining, then the birth-rate will tend to decline even more during a period of postponement. The reduction in the norm may be looked upon as contributing permanent postponements. This may have happened to some extent since 1970. Alternatively a decline in the norm may tend to dampen the rise in the birth-rate during a period of advancement and acceleration of family building. It may well be that the rise in the birth-rate after 1955, steep though it was, would have been even steeper had the norm of family size not begun to fall.

Since the birth-rate is the ratio of live births to the total population, male and female, old and young, married and non-married, fertile and non-fertile alike, changes in the structure of the population will affect the birth-rate quite apart from changes in the pace of family building. If the proportion of older people in the population is increased, as happened after 1910 when the annual number of births began to fall steeply, the denominator of the birth-rate is increasingly inflated by those who are no longer capable of contributing to the numerator. The rate itself is therefore deflated and any decline in the birth-rate is accentuated. Conversely a persistent rise in the birth-rate will, within fifteen years or so, begin to increase the proportion of fertile women in the total population and to reduce the non-fertile proportion, and this will tend to inflate the birth-rate. This, too, has occurred since 1970.

Finally, a decline in foetal mortality (and there has been a progressive reduction in the stillbirth-rate, especially since 1960) will increase the proportion of pregnancies that result in live births and will tend to raise the birth-rate. Other mortality changes may work in the opposite direction. For example, if more people survive to older ages, this has the effect of increasing the proportion of old people in the population, i.e. of deflating the birth-rate.

Changes in the timing of family building are therefore not always reflected in changes in the birth-rate as clearly as they would otherwise be, because of these overlying influences of changes in the family size norm, in population structure and in mortality.

When we come to consider the annual number of live births in the country, the size of the population and especially the number of women within the reproductive age range become additional factors. The more women there are who are making a contribution to family building in a particular year, the more babies there will be even though the family size norm and the timing pattern remains unchanged. Moreover, changes in the annual number of births become, some fifteen years later, changes in the number of women at risk, so to speak, of motherhood. So without any implications for changes in family size a peak or hump in the annual number of births in any year or group of years (for example in 1955−64) would be expected, other things being equal, to be echoed fifteen to twenty years later (say in 1975−84). Things are rarely equal. If births are postponed either temporarily or permanently, the echo may be delayed or diminished (it did not in fact occur until 1978). But, let us repeat, the echoing rise in the annual number of births would hold no implication for change in the norm of family size.

To sum up, changes in the birth-rate or in the annual number of births have very little to do with the real level of fertility, i.e. the size of family ultimately produced by a woman by the end of her reproductive age period. To describe every continued rise in the weekly number of births as a baby boom and every continued fall as a baby famine, as the newspapers tend to do, is very misleading.

Period Total Fertility Rate

For the same reasons that lead us to reject the crude birth-rate as a measure of fertility level, we must also reject another measure which seems to be popular, namely the period total fertility rates. This is the total of the age specific fertility rates (usually in five-year age groups) in a particular period, usually a calendar year. It looks like a figure of average family size and it is indeed the number of children a woman would have if she proceeded through a reproductive life having children year by year and age by age at the rates recorded for women of each age in one specific year. But these rates are the contributions to total family building of women of different marriage cohorts at different stages of their reproductive life in that one particular calendar year. The rate is therefore just as likely to be distorted by changes in the timing of family building as the crude birth-rate. For example if in 1979 young women are postponing births (which they intend to have later), and older women have already finished their family building, then all the age rates will be lowered (even if the family size norm has remained unchanged) and the period total fertility rate will be much lower than the average family size which successive cohorts will actually produce. Something like this has been happening in many European countries in recent years. Between 1970 and 1975 the following changes were observed. (Table I).

Table I
Period total fertility rate

	1970	1975
Federal Republic of Germany	2·1	1·4
France	2·5	1·9
Great Britain	2·4	1·8
Netherlands	2·6	1·8

In 1970 the family size norm in Great Britain may not have been very different from 2·4, but in 1975 it had not fallen as low as 1·8. Late in 1977 it appeared that the most recent spell of postponement had come to an end, and if this is true it is likely that the age specific fertility rates of young ages will cease to be deflated while on the other hand the rates at higher ages will be inflated by make-up births. The period total fertility rate will then be inflated possibly to a value above the family size norm. Indeed the period total fertility rate which fell to as low as 1·7 in 1977 rose to 2·0 in 1978 and is still rising. The family size norm has however probably changed very little for marriages during the last twenty years. So the period total fertility rate is no guide to changes in the ultimately achieved family sizes of couples. It is this last measure, the actual achieved family size, which is the only true measure of fertility and the only reliable guide to the prospects for growth or decline of the population.

Family Size

Unmarried women are not all childless; indeed the number of single parent families is growing. But a large proportion of unmarried women are childless. To allow for this and for childhood mortality, married couples must produce families of slightly more than two children on average, if every adult in the population is to be replaced. If one considers the replacement of males separately from that of females, then allowance has to be made for the sex ratio of births (there are fewer girl than boy babies). All in all, we need for replacement an average completed family size of 2·1 live born children per woman; and this means an average of about 2·2 per *married* woman.

With this yardstick in mind, we may now look at the changes in completed families for successive marriage cohorts in Great Britain. These are shown in Table II. These figures are shown graphically in Fig. 1. When the fertility statistics of Great Britain are looked at in this longer term perspective it can be seen that there has been a persistent downward trend in family size which has continued since the latter part of the nineteenth century.

Table II
Great Britain: average completed family size (number of live born children) for marriages in different periods

Period of marriage	Average family size
1870–79	5·8
1880–89	5·1
1890–99	4·7
1900–09	3·4
1910	3·1
1915	2·5
1920	2·5
1925	2·2
1930	2·1
1935	2·1
1940	2·0
1945	2·2
1950	2·3
1955	2·4[a]
1960	2·4[a]
1965	2·3[a]

[a] Projected.

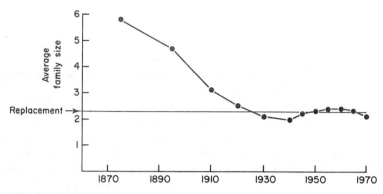

FIG. 1. England and Wales — average family size for different marriage cohorts.

Factors Affecting Changes in Family Size

The Industrial Revolution in this country, as elsewhere in Europe, was a labour-intensive expansion of economic activity. There was work for the entire family, both children and adults. The larger the family, the greater the household income. Large families, in consequence, were much in favour.

The decline in family size which began in the latter part of the nineteenth century can be explained in part by the beginning of the now familiar and all too frequent cycles of over-production followed by depression, retrenchment and unemployment which led to much poverty. However, it is explained mainly by the enactment of the Shaftesbury legislation prohibiting the employment of young children and the Elementary Education Act of 1870 which made attendance at primary school compulsory from the age of five to 13. Almost overnight, young children ceased to be economic assets to their parents and became economic liabilities.

A further dramatic change took place at the turn of the century as a consequence of a sharp decline in infant mortality. This was brought about by the 1875 Public Health Act and by specialized maternity and child welfare centres. The first health visitors' training courses began in 1892. At the beginning of the century a number of towns had milk depots for the provision of clean cows' milk for poor mothers unable to breastfeed their infants. These and similar agencies formed the foundation of the maternity and child welfare service as we know it today. In addition to this concentration on the health of mothers and babies, social conditions were generally improving. As a result infant mortality (deaths under one year of age per 100 live births), which had been above 150 throughout the latter half of the nineteenth century, fell from 156 in the period 1896−1900 to 90 for the period 1916−1920 and 55 for 1936−40. There was a new confidence in the survival of infants. It was no longer necessary, as it had been in Victorian times, to think in terms of producing six or seven children in order that five should survive to adult life.

All these influences taken together, but especially the economic influences, brought about a profound change of attitude to family size: a swift progression to a smaller norm. For the poorer circumstanced the norm remained higher than for the better circumstanced, but in all levels of society smaller families became the order of the day.

It is important to recognize that in the face of lack of access to contra-ceptives*, the change in public attitude, though not necessarily coherent or articulate, must have been resolute.

What we have been seeing then is a long trend towards an average family size of about replacement level. Reaction to the great economic depression brought the average family size below replacement level (and probably below the true norm in terms of social attitudes) for those married between 1925 and 1935. Wartime conditions kept the average family size low for later marriages. After World War II there was some recovery and, more recently still, it appears that for those married in the "you never had it so good" era of the late 1950s, the average family size will turn out to be slightly above replacement requirements (Cartwright, 1976).

The Prospective Trend

The recovery in fertility exhibited by marriages of the late 1950s and early 1960s would appear to be as short-lived as the economic euphoria which may have prompted it. Attitudes favouring small families have been hardening.

In 1967 the Office of Population Censuses and Surveys (OPCS)

---

* "Everyone is aware of the prolonged decline of fertility in most industrialised countries between the 1870's and the 1930's but it is perhaps not quite so widely realized that this decline owed little to modern technology. The vulcanization of rubber and, later, the use of liquid latex, were important to the development of mechanical contraception. But the primary means of control was coitus interruptus, supplemented, to an extent which probably differed between different countries by illegal abortions. This was still largely the case in the 1930's and 1940's." D.V. Glass (1976).

carried out a survey of attitudes to family size (Woolf, 1971) in a representative sample of married women in Great Britain. Table III summarizes the responses of this sample to a question about the number of children they expected to have.

Table III
Family Intention Survey 1967. All ages of wife: average expected number of children

Date of marriage	Minimum	Most likely	Maximum
Before 1945	2·7	2·7	2·8
1945−49	2·4	2·5	2·6
1950−54	2·4	2·7	2·8
1955−59	2·2	2·7	2·8
1960−64	1·9	2·5	2·8
1965 or later	1·7	2·5	2·9

It will immediately be noted that the 'most likely' figure of 2·5 for the marriages of 1945−49 is higher than the actual figure of 2·3 shown in Table II, so the figures may be biased in an upward direction. But certainly the 'most likely' figure is lower for marriages of 1960 or later than for marriages of 1950−59.

The survey was repeated in 1972 (for the same sample) (Woolf and Pegden, 1976) with the response shown in Table IV. The authors feel that more confidence can be placed on these later figures because, as a result of changes of view following experience with children and pressures of married life, "the numbers of children a woman expects to have may be more validly and reliably assessed some four to five years after marriage rather than at marriage, and particular emphasis should be placed on the views of women who at that time have two children". They go on to say: "If then the number of children these women expect to have in 1972 — after five but less than 13 years of marriage — are studied they suggest a mean number of 2·3 children expected altogether". However the authors are here averaging all marriages recent and less recent. Table IV suggests that for marriages of the late 1960s the average family size will be 2·1.

During 1976 the General Household Survey of the Office of Population Censuses and Surveys introduced, in England and Wales, a question to married women about family size. These women were asked about the number expected at marriage, the number actually born at the time of interview and number expected at the time of interview. Table V summarizes the results.

These figures confirm the finding of Woolf and Pegden that in the

Table IV
Family Intention Survey 1972

Date of Marriage	Mean number of children ideal for couples "like yourselves" in 1972
1960−61	2·3
1962−63	2·2
1964−65	2·1
1966−67	2·1

case of incomplete families expectations are lowered after a few years of maternal experience. They also confirm their finding that for marriages after 1965 the average expected family size may be as low as 2·1. The final column of Table IV does suggest a downward trend. It would appear that the prospects are of a period of below replacement fertility. How long this period may be depends on what happens to a number of factors which may affect fertility.

Marriage

Although the proportion of births which are classified as illegitimate has risen from 4·7 per cent in 1951−55 to 8·7 per cent in 1971−75 and 9·2 per cent in 1976, it still remains true that most births are born in marriage and that marriage rates exercise a powerful influence on the level of fertility. Age of marriage is also important since though most couples now exercise fertility control, the younger the age of marriage of a woman, the longer the period during which she is at risk of conception. After the sharp fall from 1946 to 1970 the average age at marriage has remained low though it has risen very slightly. The median age, which is less affected by late marriages, has remained steady for women at 21·4 years. The annual rate of first marriage for women per 1000 single

Table V
General Household Survey 1976. Average number of children expected

Year of present marriage	Expected at marriage	Born at interview	Expected at interview
Pre 1960	2·4	2·6	2·6
1960−64	2·3	2·3	2·3
1965−69	2·3	1·9	2·1
1970−74	2·0	0·9	1·9

females aged 16 and over, after rising from 75·7 in 1946−50 to 98·6 in 1970 has fallen as the figures in Table VI indicate.

Table VI
England and Wales: first marriages per 1000 single females aged 16 and over

1970	98·6
1971	96·2
1972	97·3
1973	90·9
1974	85·8
1975	83·5
1976	76·8

This reduction applies to all individual age groups under 45. If this fall persists it will lead to a fall in the proportion of spinsters who marry before reaching the end of their reproductive life. The proportion of married women who married before age 45 among the generation born in 1900 was 84 per cent. This has risen to the very high value of 95 per cent, for those born in 1930, the last generation for which it is currently possible to make this calculation (Office of Population Censuses and Surveys, 1978). A fall in the proportion will mean, other things being equal, that those who do marry will have to produce larger families than formerly required for replacement to make up for the shortfall in marriages. It means that the average family size of 2·1 in prospect for those who marry will be even less sufficient for replacement.

Birthplace of Mother

In 1971 at a duration of marriage of 15−19 completed years (i.e. married approximately 1951−55) the average family size of women born in the West Indies was 3·4, in the Indian subcontinent 3·5, and in the Irish Republic 2·8, as compared with 2·3 for all birthplaces taken together. However this represents early experience among immigrants. There are clear signs that fertility rates have fallen in recent years−very substantially so for West Indian born women (Office of Population Censuses and Surveys, 1978). It is common experience that immigrants quickly adapt to the fertility norms of their host countries. Immigrant women (within the limits of their religious background) are as strongly motivated towards rearing smaller families as their native compatriots and for the same reasons. It seems unlikely that any excess in immigrant as compared with native fertility will be a factor in arresting the present decline. The figures of all preceding tables in this paper include immigrants.

Social Class and Socio-Economic Groups

The long decline in fertility has affected all social classes, but the average size of family in Social Class V (unskilled manual workers) has remained consistently higher than in Social Class I (professional workers). However there has been a recent change in the pattern of social class differences. Between 1911 and 1951 there was a steady gradient in average family size rising from Social Class I to Social Class V. In 1961, and even more so in 1971, the gradient became U-shaped, the lowest average family size being found in Social Class III (skilled non-manual workers). Table VII shows figures from the 1951 and 1971 censuses.

Table VII
Average number of live-born children to women in their first marriage

Census	I Professional	II Intermediate (including most managerial and senior admin.)	III Skilled		IV Partly-skilled manual	V Unskilled
1951 Completed fertility (women aged 45−49 at census)	1·51	1·62	1·93		2·36	2·64
1971			IIIN Non-Manual	IIIM Manual		
Duration 15−19 years i.e. married approximately 1951−55	2·26	2·18	2·02	2·37	2·40	2·74

Despite this new disturbance in the social gradient, it still seems likely that, in the main, any future social mobility in an upward direction will tend to depress the overall fertility level.

Education

Social class is an indication of the overall level of living including many elements — housing, nutrition, health care, education, leisure, etc. One of these elements, education, has been shown in previous census analyses to have an influence upon fertility. Generally, the higher the age at which full-time education ceases (for both husband and wife), the lower the average family size. Here again there has been some departure from this simple relationship. While those with minimal secondary education (terminal education age 15 or under) have larger families than those who left school before the age of 19 (and this applies to husbands and wives independently), it appears that for marriages during the period of fertility recovery of the 1950s, average family size, where both parents remained in full-time education until age 20 or later, was almost as high as those with minimal education. It did become fashionable at that time for those in professional and academic occupations to have families of three or four children and this may go some way to explaining the disturbance in the social gradient previously remarked upon. It should be borne in mind that this group represents a small minority with proportionately diminished influence upon the overall level of fertility in this country. Generally it remains true that any raising of the average terminal age of education will tend to reduce the average size of family.

As to the mechanism of this association, it is possible that the more educated parents are more knowledgeable and more effective in controlling their fertility, but it is also likely that there is a link with the full-time employment of the mother and the motivation for fertility control that this supplies, i.e. that more of the educated women are in professional or managerial careers that lead them to be more resolute in limiting their families.

Employment

Information from the 1976 General Household Survey shows that the average family size for women married in 1960—64 at ages under 30 and who were in paid employment in the week prior to interview was about 2·1 compared with nearly 2·6 for those who were not working. This is simply a gross differential for all kinds of employment taken together and it is probable that some women could not enter paid employment *because* they had families (rather than vice versa). But paradoxically in a period of economic depression and of high unemployment, the proportion of married women who are in full-time paid employment is still increasing and exceeds one half. Therefore any depressive effect on fertility arising from the full-time employment of married women seems likely to increase.

Other Factors

The present low level of fertility is not due solely to the influence of economic factors. The Federal Republic of Germany is the most prosperous and vigorous economy in Europe; it has also the lowest level of fertility. To a greater or lesser degree in different individuals there is, in the background to attitudes to family building, much concern for the conflicts arising from the pressure of world population growth and economic advancement of the developing countries on limited world resources — especially, but not only, on energy resources. There is concern for the political conflicts arising from economic difficulties within individual countries, especially those where poverty and wealth, under-consumption and over-production coexist — conflicts which tend to spill across national boundaries. Concern for the threat not only of nuclear war but of individual nuclear disaster. Concern for the conservation of the environment against the encroachment of perpetual 'economic growth'. Concern for the quality of life — for space, for health, for cultural expression, for freedom — all of which seem so much more threatened than at the beginning of this century.

Implications

While these concerns remain uneased there is not likely to be any recovery of fertility from what would appear to be a lower than replacement level. Moreover there seems to be little prospect of the present extremely high level of unemployment being substantially reduced in less than several years. Meanwhile other low fertility factors — the extension of secondary education, the extension of woman's choice of role in society, some slackening in marriage rates, the assimilation of immigrant groups — persist. All in all, there is the prospect of a period of a below replacement level of fertility for current and future marriages lasting longer than that which affected marriages between 1930 and 1940. The annual number of births in Great Britain will continue to rise for several years, partly because some postponed births may be currently being made up and partly because the women of the larger generations of 1955 – 65 are now passing through their reproductive lives. The annual number of births will then decline sharply. The temporary rise will not be an indication of anything happening to a woman's total lifetime fertility: the newspapers will call it a baby boom (perhaps in the hope of enlarging it), but it will conceal a depression.

References

Cartwright, Ann (1976). *How Many Children?* London: Routledge & Kegan Paul.
Glass, D.V. (1976). Recent and prospective trends in fertility in developed countries. *Philosophical Transactions*, **274B**, 9.
Office of Population Censuses and Surveys (1978). *Demographic Review, Great Britain: 1977*, Series DR No. 1. London: HMSO.
Woolf, M. (1971). *Family Intentions*. London: HMSO.
Woolf, M. and Pegden, S. (1976). *Families Five Years On*. London: HMSO.

Fertility Policies in the Latin American Continent

B. VIEL

International Planned Parenthood Federation, London, England

It is impossible to understand the present Latin American demographic problem without referring, albeit briefly, to the history of the continent.

Considerable numbers of studies have tried to estimate the population of Latin America at the time the Conquerors arrived. The most recent estimations indicate that 100 million is a very probable figure — about 25 million in what is today Mexico and probably a little over ten million in what is today Peru, the former Inca Empire. The rest were scattered around the vast continent in groups ranging from those who were extremely primitive, living only from hunting, to groups that practised very primitive agriculture.

In spite of the high level of development achieved in the Mexican and Incan Empires, neither of these civilisations had developed the wheel. Since no animals could be used for transportation except a small member of the camel family in the highlands of the Andean region, it can be said that the only source of energy that pre-Colombian man had was human muscle. No doubt at that time the whole population of the continent was pro-natalistic. What happened with the arrival of the Conquerors is shown by numerical evidence from Mexico and Peru. A hundred years after the arrival of Hernán Cortes in Mexico a population that had been around 25 million had been reduced to only one million. A similar depopulation occurred in Peru. The reasons for such a demographic catastrophe are multiple. Apparently the most important was the impact of new diseases brought by the Spaniards, to which the native population had no natural resistance, among them measles, smallpox, enteric infections, etc. Furthermore, the disruption of the life of the natives contributed to the maintenance of a very high death-rate for many years. What had been a chiefly agricultural society was changed. Men were sent to the mines as slaves and the great plains were converted into cattle-raising lands. Such massive changes had a profound effect on nutrition and fertility.

Since the Spaniards went to America to become land-owners and not to work with their hands, the depopulation of the natives was an unexpected blow to their ambitions. The vast territory that they had conquered had insufficient human beings to labour in it. The need for more and more human beings in a continent in which the native population was dying out and in which a very small minority of Europeans, mainly Spaniards and Portuguese, were land-owners, led to the mixture of races and a sort of polygamy in which the Conquerors themselves mixed with the surviving native women and encouraged the same practice among the native groups. The whole population of Latin America was encouraged to reproduce itself in the same way that the cattle owners encouraged the reproduction of their animals.

The high death-rate prevented success, and the only solution was forced migration from Africa, a repulsive slave trade that lasted until Independence at the beginning of the nineteenth century and persisted in Brazil up to the year 1870. Since the negro African adapted better to the tropical regions of Latin America, most of the slave trade was concentrated in the lands that were suitable for the production of sugar and cotton, the main tropical products that could be exported to Europe.

In spite of the strong pro-natalist policy during the 300 years of the Colonial period, the total population of Latin America at the time of Independence was still lower than that estimated at the time of the arrival of the Spaniards. The European colonizers, the vast slave trade and the numbers of those born in the continent, were not enough to compensate for the very high death-rate prevalent during the whole Colonial period.

Between 1810 and 1820 those who were white or had a high percentage of white ancestry were the land-owners with economic but no political power. All the political power belonged to the Spaniards born in the Peninsula who were sent to America as administrators of the Colony. When Napoleon invaded Spain, the pretext was ready and Latin America began its War of Independence. After a long and cruel fight Latin America became completely independent from Spain with the exception of Cuba and Puerto Rico, which were liberated later in the century. The vast empire was divided into small countries, most of which fell into a long period of chaotic anarchy. Wars between them as well as internal guerrilla warfare and revolutions designed to seize power lasted for many years in several of the new countries.

During the Colonial period the Church provided almost the only route for social mobility for those born out of the local land-owning aristocracy. After the War of Independence a new way was opened, the

Army. Anyone could become a General and acquire political and economic power. It was only very late in the nineteenth century that the liberal professions began to open a third way, giving rise to the intellectual middle class. Militarism was inherited with Independence and still prevails. For the common people the independence obtained did not mean a great change. The slaves were freed, but the system of very small salaries was maintained and labour forces lived in almost the same extremely poor conditions as during the Colonial period.

The pro-natalist policy did not change at all. The continent was still extremely underpopulated with a need for more human beings to carry out the daily work, added to the demand for more soldiers for the armies that were dividing the continent into the different countries that exist today. Between Independence and 1920 almost no improvement in the environment took place. The cities were as unsafe as mediaeval cities in Europe and the condition of those living in rural areas was no better. The birth-rate in most countries was as high as 50 per thousand, but the death-rate was almost as high and the natural increase could be estimated at no higher than one half per cent per year. In the year 1920 it is estimated that the total population of the continent was no more than 90 million, still lower than the estimated total population at the time of the Conquest, in spite of the fact that certain regions — those that had achieved peace and political stability earlier than others — received a flood of migration from Europe. The southern part of the continent — Argentina, Uruguay and to a lesser degree Chile — received from the middle of the nineteenth century to the First World War many European migrants. The same can be said of the southern region of Brazil. Up to 1920 Latin America was chiefly a continent living on its mines and agriculture. The First World War forced Latin America to begin industrialization, together with an increasing movement towards urbanization, but still the death-rate was sufficiently high to prevent natural increase higher than one per cent per year. Had a demographer attempted in 1920 to predict the future population of the continent based on the natural growth existing at that period, he would have said that Latin America would have a population of 180 million by the year 1990.

At the end of the thirties, sulpha drugs were discovered. Around 1945 DDT became available to control malaria without draining the swamps. By 1950 antibiotics were in use. Owing to these technological advances which were imported into the continent, the death-rate that had been as high as 30 per thousand dropped in a very short period to an average of eight per thousand. The birth-rate remained high, fluctuating between 45 per thousand in the tropical regions and 35 per thousand in the colder areas of the continent. The Latin American demographic explosion had begun and a continent that in around 1920 had a natural growth of one per cent per year, reached a natural growth of three per cent per year, a percentage rarely observed in the whole history of humanity.

The governments on the whole did not react to the new conditions. The pro-natalist policy of the Colonial period, carefully maintained during the first 140 years of Independence, was not changed at all in the face of the new developments. Those who observed what was happening with this explosive increase in population were not alarmed. They thought that the phenomenon had natural laws that would take care of it and the experience of the European continent was invoked to maintain the view that what had happened in Europe would also happen in Latin America. It was assumed that according to demographic transition theory the decline in the death-rate would later give rise to a decline in the birth-rate and that the natural growth would tend to diminish spontaneously through the years until it reached the low level that is now observed in Europe. For most of the governments there was no reason for concern.

During the last thirty years the continent has increased its population to a figure at present estimated at 350 million. Even if a small decline in the average birth-rate of the continent is achieved, it would be extremely difficult by the end of the century for the total population of Latin America to be less than 620 million. Certainly demographic transition theory is not applicable universally. Even in Europe it cannot be said that it has operated uniformly. Occidental Europe experienced a spontaneous decline in the birth-rate that was not observed in Eastern Europe at a similar level until contraception and abortion were available. Even within Occidental Europe, France and Ireland are good examples that demographic transition theory does not always apply. Ireland still has a higher birth-rate than the rest of Europe, while in the last 180 years France has not seen a period in which the birth-rate greatly exceeded the death-rate. Declines in both have been perfectly parallel.

In the Latin American continent, with the exception of Argentina and Uruguay, countries almost entirely populated by European migrants, demographic transition theory has not applied at all. Death-rates have been declining substantially since 1940 and, owing to the extreme youth of the populations are now lower overall than the rate prevailing in Europe. In spite of this decline the birth-rate is still very high, and only a few countries exhibit a decline in birth-rate over the last ten years. The decline observed chiefly in Costa Rica, Panama, Colombia and Chile is coincident with strong family planning programmes and an increased number of women who year by year resort to contraceptive practices. Probably the most dramatic decline in the birth-rate is that observed in Chile, where it dropped from 35 per thousand in 1964 to 22 per thousand in 1978. Such a decline is in perfect accord with the increasing percentage of women using methods to control their fertility. To date, 25 per cent of women of reproductive age are using reversible contraceptives and about 12 per cent of women of reproductive age have been surgically sterilized.

In the rest of the Latin American continent there are no signs yet of a decline in the birth-rate and the population is still growing at an average estimated rate of 2·8 per cent per year. Some governments, though tolerant of private efforts, do not support any large-scale programme of family planning. Others maintain the pro-natalist policy of the earlier period and go as far as to consider illegal the information and distribution of contraceptive methods.

Fortunately one of the strongest pro-natalist governments, that of the large country Mexico, has reversed its policy in the last two years and the government now supports a family planning programme that it is hoped will succeed, but it is still too soon to evaluate results. In Brazil, the largest country in the continent, the population already numbering 110 million is still increasing at the rate of 2·8 per thousand, yet the government continues to maintain a strong pro-natalist policy.

It appears that demographic transition theory operated only in Argentina and Uruguay. The decline in Costa Rica, Panama, Colombia and Chile has not been spontaneous and is coincident with the programmes supported by the governments. Mexico did not show any sign of decline until its government decided to offer contraception and sterilization. The present government of Cuba, which at the beginning maintained that there was no such thing as a population problem and that by arranging a better distribution of income the birth-rate would come down spontaneously, is now conducting a family planning programme, offering free services of contraception, sterilization and abortion. Since the introduction of these measures the birth-rate in Cuba has begun to decline.

Problems

As was to be expected, the sudden and enormous demographic explosion in the Latin American continent created a series of severe economic and social problems. A continent that in general was an exporter of food is now importing it, in spite of the fact that its agricultural output has increased to nearly four times that of thirty years ago. Despite the increase in agricultural production and the increasing quantity of food obtained from abroad, it is estimated now that nearly 30 per cent of children under five suffer from some form of malnutrition.

The illiteracy rate expressed as a percentage has diminished but the increased number of young people has overtaken the increase in educational facilities and the total number of illiterate people is now greater than it was 30 years ago. Industrialization has increased considerably and urbanization is now a common feature of the continent. Around 1950 only 30 per cent of the population was urban. Today the figure is over 60 per cent and in certain countries it is already 80 per cent. The speed of growth of the cities has been such that it has been impossible to build enough houses and to provide them with a reliable water supply and sewage system. In all the big cities of Latin America there is a marginal population that lives without what is regarded as minimal environmental protection, and which has to live in very dangerous and overcrowded conditions. Disease is prevalent and if the death-rate is low, it is only due to successful treatment of infection.

A continent that during the whole Colonial period and the first 150 years of Independence was dreaming of a larger population, now finds itself with such vast numbers that it is unable to provide its people with minimal conditions of sanitation, unable to give them even a minimal education, and probably worst of all, unable to offer them work. In order to produce more food agricultural production has been mechanized and a large number of rural workers have become unemployed. The so-called 'green revolution' is producing more food with less workers.

The industrial movement is taking advantage of the most modern machines imported from the developed world. The more modern they are, the fewer workers they need. Those who hoped that industry was going to provide enough jobs for the increasing population now find that it is entirely unable to absorb the increasing number of young people looking for work. Unemployment, together with under-employment, are reaching percentages as high as 30 to 40 per cent of the active population. The social unrest resulting from such a dangerous situation can easily be guessed.

In spite of such severe social and economic problems, the majority of governments are still indifferent to (when not totally against) measures designed to diminish the speed of growth of the population. The effects of family planning programmes will be seen in 20 to 30 years from now. Those in power are sure that they will not be members of the government at that time and prefer to secure their position in office for the present, offering something that will be tangible in a short period of time. Building a factory, a bridge, a hospital or a school is much more popular and appealing to them than promoting a family planning programme.

Governments reluctant to see the reality and to estimate the magnitude of the demographic catastrophe that will be observed in the next few years are heavily supported by the upper hierarchy of the Catholic Church and by the Marxist political parties. The upper hierarchy of the Church claims that contraceptive methods are against natural law. The Marxist parties clearly see that the increasing rate of unemployment will produce a revolution in which they will be the winners; family planning for them is a morphine that delays the pressure for changing the system. They claim that they will accept anti-natalist policies as soon as they are in power, together with all the other changes that the Marxist regime implies, but they are not ready to accept it in isolation. If they attain the power they are seeking they will discover that, unfortunately, the speed of growth of the population cannot suddenly be stopped and that they will be in a very difficult position, trying to solve the problems of unemployment, undernourishment and illiteracy in a population that has increased beyond the capability of the existing resources to sustain it.

If governments with few exceptions have been indifferent or opposed to efforts to control population growth, the women have been uniformly in favour of regulating their fertility. Knowing no other way, they have resorted to illegal abortion, which is now reaching epidemic proportions throughout the continent. A conservative estimate of the number of illegal abortions performed in one year is at the level of six million. With rare uniformity, all the hospitals in Latin America are reporting that about 30 per cent of the obstetrical beds are occupied by cases who suffer complications resulting from illegal abortion performed by untrained hands, when not self-induced. This epidemic of illegal abortions is one of the most appalling social injustices in the continent. Those who have money obtain safe abortions from professionals who know how to perform the operation; those who are poor and cannot afford the cost of a safe abortion have to risk their lives by resorting to very unsafe techniques.

All the epidemiological studies done in relation to illegal abortion prove that 80 per cent of women hospitalized because of complications are married or common law wives between 20 and 30 years of age who have already had three or more children; they are using abortion from a sense of responsibility towards the children they have already had. In my own experience in a Chilean hospital 80 per cent of the victims of the complications of illegal abortion claim to be Catholic.

Opinion surveys in all the Latin American countries differ very little about what women consider is the ideal family size. The majority of answers give three children as the number desired, only a very small minority still answer the survey with the traditional teaching of the Church: "as many as God wills".

Now we see a continent in which there are countries with a birth-rate of 45 per thousand, such as Honduras, Guatemala, El Salvador and others with birth-rates of 20 to 22 per thousand such as Argentina, Chile, Cuba and Uruguay. Such differences when the great majority of women of all these countries have expressed their desire for small families, are difficult to explain. The great variety of explanations put forward are based on loose assumptions and a very small amount of scientific research. The easiest answer is to attribute the differences observed among the countries to economic development. Argentina is a rich country, Honduras is a very poor one. Argentina has a birth-rate of 20 per thousand, Honduras one of 45. Those who use such arguments forget that the richest country in the continent is Venezuela, whose birth-rate is over 37 per thousand.

There is a very clear correlation between the percentage of illiterate people and the birth-rate; the higher the incidence of illiteracy, the higher the birth-rate. It would be easy to conclude that education is the answer, forgetting that among those hospitalized because of illegal abortion there are many illiterate people.

Personally I am convinced that it is impossible to isolate one factor. It is easy to see that the number of children per woman diminishes in inverse ratio to the number of years spent in the educational system. Women with a university education have an average of two children, while women with incomplete primary education have four and the illiterate have five or more, but the level of education expresses much more than the education itself. University education means a higher income, proper housing and access to all kinds of facilities to regulate fertility. Illiteracy means a very low income, no work and no facilities unless the government provides them.

In conclusion, I am convinced that the birth-rate declines proportionally to the increase in the percentage of women practising effective contraceptive methods. Such a percentage depends on the facilities that the government organizes to allow the poorer sections of the community to obtain contraception that the well-to-do obtain from the private medical profession and pharmaceutical stores.

THE GALTON LECTURE

The Centrality of Demographic Experience

PETER LASLETT

Cambridge Group for the History of Population and Social Structure, Cambridge, England

Previous Galton Lecturers may have been from Trinity College, Cambridge, and Francis Galton was himself a member of that college. It seems probable, however, that few historians have had the honour of delivering the Galton Lecture, and certainly none from the Cambridge Group for the History of Population and Social Structure.

The centrality of demographic experience may appear to be a rather unexpected theme in a symposium devoted to changing patterns of conception and fertility. Yet its content of fertility and its history is indeed relevant, perhaps in a rather unexpected way. Recent investigation into the history of conception and fertility, much of which (in the case of England at least) has been done by Wrigley and Schofield at Cambridge, has produced remarkable results which have taken well over a decade to obtain and then only through the joint efforts of scores of part-time researchers all over the country as well as from the work at Cambridge. The tradition of investigation which they represent goes back a long way in the intellectual history of Britain, certainly to Rickman, the founder of British censuses; to Malthus, perhaps the greatest figure in the history of the study of population; even to Petty, Graunt and King, the English pioneers of historical demography, of econometrics and of historical sociology as a whole. It would have pleased them, as it would certainly have pleased Francis Galton, to know that there would come a time when surprisingly accurate and fairly complete information would become available on the demographic history of our country over the whole period of its industrial transformation, information which preoccupied them so much and which they found it impossible to establish.

The phrase 'the centrality of demographic experience' is not necessarily an assertion that demographic experience *must* be taken as central for the individual, central for the study of society. Indeed, the very terms themselves are to some extent question-begging. For centrality is a metaphor, and no more than this. It is certainly a suggestive metaphor,

23

and one which is evidently found intellectually satisfying, a metaphor of social relationships monarchically arranged. One can question, however, the assumption that social reality need be centrally organized at all, or if it is so, why that centre should be singular, not plural. One can try to decide where demography would fit into a social world poly-archically arranged, or into one in which both principles were in some way combined. Issues such as these are undoubtedly complex, such queries can be raised, but can be left there.

In the most general sense, a claim that demographic experience is central amounts to no more than the assertion that the word demo-graphic here refers to the recording and analysis of events which are enormously important to the persons to whom they happen. We are all born, a very large proportion of us gets married, and we are all destined to die. Because each of these events is of high salience for all human beings and for their associates, relatives and friends, even for their enemies, demography is inevitably central to experience, social experience as well as individual experience. We can assume further-more, perhaps with some marginal uncertainty, that all our prede-cessors had identical attitudes, and all our successors will do so too. Demography so defined, therefore, is central to drama and to literature, even to that species of literature which is my special concern — history — history as a muse.

A history which failed to recognize the centrality of demographic experiences in this sense, and which failed to make use of demographic analysis in the process of observing, discussing and reflecting upon past individuals and past societies, would have two shortcomings. One would be an imperfection, an avoidable imperfection, in its grasp of what happened to these people and to their society, and the other would be a failure in sympathy. Not only would such a history pass over the effects of demographic events, in limiting and to some degree determining their behaviour, as people and as a society; it would also be indifferent to their anxieties and their aspirations about themselves. A want of under-standing, a want in sensitivity, a want in respect for those past persons as persons, would be unforgivable. It is the duty of the historian to observe individuals going about their business in the past knowing infinitely less about them than their contemporaries knew, and than they knew about themselves. But about one thing of supreme importance to each and all of them is that he has privileged awareness. He knows when they were going to die, and this makes each of his subjects into the protagonist of a personal tragedy. Such knowledge gives something of a god-like quality to historical reflection.

The same attribute, if nothing like the same realism, that realism which gives to historical writing its peculiar fascination, attaches to all imaginative literature. Dramatists and novelists know what is going to happen to their characters because they have made it all up already. But they have to make sure that what they have made up is about demographic experience, and believable demographic experience at that, or else they will neither be listened to nor read.

These considerations about literature and history read like truisms. Once recognized they may seem too tedious to dwell upon, and we may be inclined to conclude that in this, its vaguest sense, the centrality of demographic experience has little analytic interest.

However, once the historian, or the reader of literature, acquires even a little principled demographic knowledge, the prospect changes. To know that only a handful of the girls alive in England when Romeo and Juliet was composed could possibly have married at age 13, that most of them were ten years older at their weddings, and had been physically incapable at Juliet's age, adds meaning to Shakespeare's dramatic purposes. To be aware, from the knowledge made available by Wrigley and Schofield, that when Jane Austen was on her deathbed in 1817, at the age of 41, she was indeed dying before her time, since her life might have been expected to continue for 25 or even 30 years longer, and that, therefore, we could well have had those unwritten works of her maturity which we should so much like to read, intensifies our detached and privileged historian's hindsight. My object in what follows is to try to show that when stricter senses of the phrase we are considering are also taken into account, its centrality shines out in unexpected and intriguing ways (Laslett, 1976).

Marriage and Family

But before giving an example which may convince you of this, there are two issues which have to be raised. One is about the status of marriage itself, and the other the question of whether demography can be called experiential at all, whether the phrase 'demographic experience' is in fact permissible.

Let us consider this point first. There are those who maintain that "demography is an analysis of indices, like cardiography, and one can have a cardiographic record, but not (usually) a cardiographic experience."* In response to such a challenge we may notice how much

---

* I quote here from a letter from Dr Jonathan Benthall, Director of the Royal Anthropol-

more easily described as experiences are the demographic vicissitudes which occur to a collectivity than those which occur to the individuals of which a collectivity is composed. We assert quite naturally that the inhabitants of the Indian sub-continent *experienced* that fall in mortality in the early twentieth century which ensured that their numbers should be so vast today. We may well allow it to be appropriate to say that an Indian mother who has given birth seven or eight times since 1950, lost one child as a baby and lost her husband too, has undergone a demographic experience, even a series of them. But we should be more inclined to pronounce that she underwent repeated parturition and bereavement. It was India, the Indian collectivity, which had the. experience, or whose demographic experience was ever so slightly modulated by what happened to this one Indian citizen. The indices which the demographer uses, therefore, and the calculations which he performs upon them, are indices of collective experience, and it seems to me quite proper to refer to that collective experience as being itself demographic.

You will have to judge whether this implied distinction is a useful one, in view of the demographic episode which I shall discuss in due course. As for marriage in relation to birth and death, there are certainly important differences. For there can be no doubt as to the biological character of birth and death, or of their social character either: they are almost universally marked out as of high social significance by rites of passage. In this way they belong firmly with what we have come inelegantly to call the biosocial sciences. But marriage is more problematic.

Its social significance needs no elaboration: marriage is a 'central' social occurrence, whatever meaning is attached to the word. But marriage is not in itself biological, since it is distinguished from procreation, and only somewhat ambiguously related with it. Even if the concept of "onset of procreative union" (Laslett, 1979a) is substituted for marriage for the purpose of demographic analysis, such a process is still different from the point of view of the individual. It does not happen to a person willy-nilly and for biological reasons, like birth and death. You have to be procreated but you do not have to procreate: there is nothing necessary about the desire to fashion a new individual in your own image, or half-image.

ogical Institute, who was in the audience when this lecture was given. He makes the interesting suggestion that "demographic experience should be reserved for those societies which show a consciousness of, and concern for, their demographic condition, as indeed some primitive as well as advanced societies do." An attractive usage, this, and one which is very close to my present argument, but distinct from it.

Reproduction is ultimately necessary of course, for social as well as for biological reasons; the biological imperative that all populations replace themselves, the urge of all societies to persist over time. But this scarcely places demography at the centre of the institution or practice of marriage. It indicates rather that demography is peripheral, if none the less indispensable. The somewhat shaded pathway linking marriage to birth and death, then, turns out to be rather intricate and uncertain, but following it step by step as we have had to do draws attention to three other features of our subject.

The first is that there does exist a filament to connect the socially central position of marriage to the intermediate and intermediary position of demography as a whole class of events and processes. Secondly, demography stands betwixt and between in several ways: between the biological and the social, between the person, with his interests and intentions, and the plurality of persons, its shape and its policies — that is to say between the individual on the one hand and the collectivity on the other (Laslett, 1979b; Wrigley, 1978).

In the third place, this consideration of marriage brings into view the relationship of demography to the family. If not exactly central to its structure and its functioning, demographic processes are indispensably associated with the family unit. It is there that procreation usually goes forward, the activity which alone makes perpetuation possible, in a society or in a population, and the family unit is its primary agent of social reproduction as distinct from biological. Procreation can, and does, proceed outside the family to some extent, and there are agents of primary socialization other than parents and any relatives who live with them, or in close contact with them. But a nation, a culture, a class, a social group of any kind, has to rely for its perpetuation for the most part on socialization within the family unit. This it was which made me the somewhat nonconformist, academically inclining, professional Englishman which I am, instead of any other of the myriad types of human individual which, as a newborn baby, I might have become.

Once the word 'family' is pronounced, numbers of other intellectual avenues open out of the discussion of the central position of demography. We cannot linger on the way in which the family of the demographer, family as kin relationship as well as family as domestic unit, is related to the family of the psychologist, the political scientist, the literary critic, and so on. We may remark in passing that there is now, as there has nearly always been, a disposition on the part of some of them to reject the necessity of a demographically sanctioned family, especially in the sense of a unit of co-residence. Fastening on the exceptions to familial procreation and familial socialization they have described the family as historically and social structurally contingent, simply the space in which productive and class forces are in interplay, disposable at the reformer's choice. Indeed, the tendency of reformist thinkers, from Plato to Thomas More to Friedrich Engels, to fasten on the family as the obstacle which has initially to be removed, has often been commented upon. It is realistic in a sense, since it recognizes in the family the agent of internalizing a social code which to them is intolerable, though its unreality in the face of what is behaviourally possible needs no under-lining (Bertaux, 1979). Yet the known demographic record of the peoples of the world, even in the turbulent century which has led up to our own time, and even in Europe, the site of so much social discontinuity, cannot be said to bear them out.

History of English Fertility

This brings us at last to our historical – demographic episode. In the later 1870s, almost exactly a century ago, the fertility of the English population began to fall, and to fall with that finality and irreversibility which ushered in the demographic transition in our country. At about the same time, and not markedly earlier as most theories of the transition might predict, mortality began to fall as well, in the same deliberate, uninterrupted way, and expectation of life went steadily upwards. The decline in birth- and death-rates continued for seventy years without a break, though with perturbations naturally during and after the First World War. By the 1930s and '40s both fertility and mortality were at a low level, fertility at a very low level.

The baby boom after the Second World War sent up births for a time in the 1950s and 1960s. There was also some immigration of young people with families to form and families to complete. But each of these movements petered out in the 1970s, and mortality, especially infant mortality, was falling steadily all the time. England provides now a standard example of a low fertility, low mortality, low- or no-growth population with an expectation of life of above 70. We are also one of the oldest populations in the world. Oldest in the sense of having so formi-dable a community of persons amongst us who are in the later or latest phases of their lives, and oldest in the sense of everyone enjoying so prolonged a duration of living.

It is clearly the fall in fertility, not the lengthening of life, that has been responsible for the great growth in the proportion of the elderly and old. A shrinking of the relative numbers of the young always increases the relative numbers of the old, and a falling mortality has little or no effect on these proportions. This is because it usually benefits the lower age groups about as much as it does their seniors on average, though concealed in this average is the fact that the very youngest, those in the first year of life, always benefit most from a decrease in deaths. The steadily diminishing English birth-rate after the 1870s was bound in the end to make the relative numbers of the elderly grow large. But the process took fifty years to become manifest in our age structure. Not until the 1920s did the fraction of the English population who had attained the age of 60 exceed 10 per cent, a figure which had probably been approached before, but never surpassed. In France 10 per cent of the population was over 60 as early as 1821 (Laslett, 1977). From the estimates of Wrigley and Schofield, it is seen that the proportion of this age group in England was smaller throughout the nineteenth century than it had ever been before, at least since the mid-sixteenth century, and that it was not until the early twentieth century that this proportion regained the level which it had attained in the early eighteenth. We seem always to have had a markedly higher relative number of the elderly than in the developing or under-developed countries of our own day, like Brazil, India or Tunisia.

Concept of Ageing

Consider for a moment the senses of the words elderly, ageing and aged as applied to collectivities, and with the historical demographic record in mind. For these expressions are of some importance to the understanding of ourselves as we now are, as we have been, and as we shall be in the foreseeable future. We need to decide quite what we mean when we say of a population or society or a nation that it has become old.

Expectation of life in England has lengthened since the 1870s from a little over 40 to a little over 70, taking both sexes together and reckoning from birth (Pressat, 1972). We certainly conform therefore to a life-expectation connotation of a population which has rapidly grown older. Pretty well everyone alive in the England we know has an excellent chance of surviving to the full life-span, a span which, it must be noted, has not itself been extended to any great degree. But if this had been the only effect of the English population in the last 100 years, if fertility had not fallen as well, we should not now have been older in the other sense, in the proportion-of-the-elderly sense. Given constant fertility and so pronounced a rise in the expectation of life at birth, we should have had today a very much larger total population. The proportion of the elderly, however, would not be very different from what it was in the 1880s, at between 7 and 8 per cent over 60. This is not much more than a third of what we are likely to have for the rest of the twentieth century.

It is perfectly possible, as can be seen from model life tables, for a population with an expectation of life greater than 70 to have only 5 per cent or fewer over the age of 60. This is provided that its fertility is high enough, or that immigration has been going on at a sufficient pace, or a combination of the two. Such may become the actual experience of the high-growth populations of our own day like India, where mortality is now falling faster than fertility, though it is unlikely that there migration will affect the issue very much. An opposite situation, where expectation of life was lower than in England a century ago, and yet where the numbers of the elderly were quite high, is not entirely out of the question. But it must be considered exceedingly unlikely, since it could only happen where fertility was, and had been, so low that the population was declining at a threatening rate. Likely examples, perhaps combined with high levels of emigration, are provided by Venice in the late seventeenth century when more than 11 per cent of the population was over 60, and Iceland in the 1720s where the proportion was no less than 14·7 per cent (Laslett, 1977).

The facts of English demographic experience are that in the 1980s the proportion of the elderly is double that of the 1920s. A fifth of our population is now aged 60 or over and a tenth is ten years or more older than this. It must be clear that without the mortality decline that produced such a remarkable rise in expectation of life the fall in fertility that occurred would have long since caused a decrease in our numbers. Had it not been for the immigration that has taken place during the last generation or so, there would certainly have been a fall in numbers and we should certainly have been more elderly than we are today, elderly in the age-composition sense. Our present prospects go like this. Should it happen that zero-growth establishes itself as a settled feature of English society, so that we approach a stationary condition in succession to our present demographic regime, we may expect a quarter of our population to be over 60 in perpetuity, or even more. It is not a demographic necessity, of course, to suppose that the age composition of the stationary population should be precisely as Pressat suggests, with a quarter of the people over 60, but it is difficult to see how it could be very different. At the present moment it seems more likely that we shall have to reckon with what might be called a quasi-stationary population, with fluctuating fertility, with a tendency for total numbers to decrease at times and with more than a quarter — perhaps approaching a third — over the age of 60.

The two senses of elderly or old when applied to collectivities, the expectation-of-life sense and the age-composition sense, then are quite distinct, and by no means necessarily imply each other. A useful definition of old as applied to a collectivity has to combine both of these senses, though age-composition has to be given by far the greater emphasis. A society with large numbers of elderly people is necessarily an old society at the time of its description, whatever the expectation of life of its members. But one where everybody born will go on living for a long time is not therefore old, even if (though not necessarily) it is due to become so. Statements made at large about life expectation, moreover, are statements about the young and inexperienced and especially about the newborn, rather than what might be called the working and directive part of a society.

Demographers and historians of course have to qualify such statements and are quite used to calculating expectation of life at all ages, in the past as well as in the present. They now know that life expectancy at the higher ages has changed much less during the last hundred years than life expectancy at birth. An Englishman of 40 in the 1880s could expect to go on living for 80 or 85 per cent as long as an Englishman of 40 in the 1980s. This was true of a prosperous citizen of Geneva a hundred years before the 1880s, and even a proletarian in that city at that time had a prospect of living after the age of 40 about two-thirds as favourable as an American male in the 1970s. If we wish to adopt a realistic definition of an old collectivity in life expectation terms, we should perhaps accept a suggestion made by Ryder (1975). There the age at which an individual or a population generally can expect to live for ten years more is taken as the index: the more advanced the year of life when that point is reached, the older the society. We may accordingly decide that a collectivity is old when one-fifth or more of the population is over 60 years of age, and one where 70 years is the age at which expectation of life is reduced to 10 years, both sexes combined in each case. This is the definition which is implied in what follows whenever a collectivity is referred to as being old, but the compositional element will often be taken to stand for both combined.

In the 1980s, therefore, we have to recognize as Englishmen that we belong to a collectivity which can be pronounced as definitively old, on the definition which has been elaborately spelt out. If we ask why this condition is unlikely to change a great deal in the short term, or indeed in the long term, we have to reckon with the following circumstances.

Prospects

A rejuvenation at the base, through an upsurge of fertility such as occurred to some extent in the 1950s and 1960s, is certainly possible. But as we have seen, it could only lead to a substantial decrease in the proportion of the old if it were large enough, and went on for long enough, to give rise at the same time to a marked expansion in our total numbers. Perhaps there are people who would welcome a big increase in the population, but all our recent declarations and resolutions have been against it.

Once set in motion a really pronounced tendency for fertility to go up would mean that the population would grow for quite a long time. When the birth-rate did go down, a bulge would travel up through the age structure which would in due course swell the proportion of the elderly and old to an even greater extent than before the rise in fertility began, until it finally died out. Emigration would not reduce the proportions of the old, because it would be the young and the fertile who would leave. Immigration, on the other hand, could lessen the tendency towards a permanently elderly population but only by sending up our numbers once again.

The sources of such an inward flow of younger, fertile people cannot under any circumstances be sought in nations of British stock, as they used to be called, unless perhaps there were great disasters in countries like Australia and New Zealand. A catastrophe nearer home, and the only one in prospect must presumably be atomic war, would be extremely unlikely to single out the old as casualties. Furthermore it would have gruesome effects on future fertility, which must have consequences for our age-composition of a kind we can scarcely imagine. I fervently hope that we can dismiss these awful possibilities, and those which in their way would be worse, like deliberately withholding welfare from the old so as to increase their mortality: or something even less humane.

Arguments of this character very quickly lead to extreme statements and sententious pessimism. I have myself no wish to deplore the ageing of our population. On the contrary, I believe that this remarkable and evidently permanent transformation presents the greatest challenge to our generation socially, culturally — intellectually a fascinating prospect. Least of all would I want to revive the identity of the demographer as the prophet of woe, and his avocation as the gloomy science, in succession to or in company with that of the economist.

The 1930s echoed with the dire warnings of demographers, or of their propagandist followers, about the imminent decline, even the extinction of the British people. Not only were these prophets wrong about numbers, but they portrayed the ageing of the population and the old themselves in ways now regarded as much too pessimistic. This is borne out even in economics. In the United States, for example, a distinguished economist of population has recently predicted that with the "growing scarcity of young adults the 1980s will see an amelioration of the unfavourable social, political and economic conditions" of the 1970s. These conditions included mounting divorce rates, high unemployment, and a lamentable increase in suicide, not to speak of an intolerable level of inflation, all apparently to be moderated by a relative decline in the younger age groups.

Here a rhythmic tendency in the established demographic regime is being postulated, where there are swings in such variables as the ratio of the young to the old, which do not go beyond certain discoverable limits. Meanwhile it has been forecast, again for the United States, from micro-simulation exercises, that the vitally important kin ties of the elderly, those links which tend to be their only really reliable relationships with the rest of the community, will grow rather than diminish over the next twenty years (Easterlin, 1978; Hammel and Wachter, 1979). No such simulation has been undertaken as yet for the British population, but it is hoped that it will be initiated in due course. The optimism of these American researchers ends at the turn of the century. They are unwilling to predict beyond that date because of the difficulty of forecasting vital rates, but they fear that the isolation of the elderly in this sense will increase.

The intellectual fascination of exploring and reflecting upon the nature and consequences of the population of our country growing old arises in many ways. Here is a community of highly experienced, predominantly healthy and active individuals with 20 or 25 years to live at leisure, leisure which is to some extent anyway genuine ease and not a time of impoverishment, dependency and anxiety. These ripened personalities show an intellectual curiosity which is not confined in Britain to the 'grammar school leavers', although it may certainly be more restricted here than in highly educated countries like the United States. They display, furthermore, a willingness to live their life of leisure as intensely as they can. But how? And what will be the future atmosphere, the cultural tone, the spirit of a whole society, the young as well as the old, which recognizes that life will go on for far longer than it has done before and progressively less of it be filled with the drudgery of earning a living?

Questions of this kind are intriguing and in stark contrast to the somewhat chauvinistic, self-pitying attitude of those who deplore the end of population growth, the departure of youth, the decay of great nations. These voices are not yet stilled in Western Europe, and the President of France has begun to talk with one of them. The outstanding fact about the age structure of the contemporary English population is that we have no cause to think ourselves peculiarly the victim of demographic circumstance, for we are not alone.

All the North-West European nations have an age composition very similar to our own, with the partial exception of the Netherlands. Austria, Sweden, West Germany and Belgium are older than the United Kingdom. Although some of the middle and Eastern European countries are approaching our condition, and although the United States and Canada have yet to approximate to their European companions, we can lay down the following principle; Western societies, rich, free, developed societies are uniquely old societies, old in the combined sense which has been described. As far as demographic calculation goes, they are very likely to remain so.

What is more they will presumably be joined in that condition by other countries as they too undergo transition and development. There are those who claim that what we have come to call the population explosion is approaching its end, that the definitive fall in fertility following upon declining mortality and ushering in the demographic transition is already taking place in many of the developing areas of the world (Tsui and Bogue, 1978; Bogue and Tsui 1979; Demeny, 1979a,b). If this is so, then the whole world may now be on its way to a finally elderly or aged population. Indeed, if the inhabitants of the globe as a whole are to survive at all, something like this must ultimately come about.

But will it follow that, because the developing countries become like us in respect of age, they will become like us in other ways and be rich, secure and well fed, too? This is a grave and decidedly hypothetical question. It is hypothetical because the end of rapidly increasing world population is still a long way off, even if the diagnosis of falling world fertility should turn out to be correct, and because the proposition that demographic transition necessarily involves economic development has never been demonstrated. The prospect of a very elderly population living at the levels of Bangladesh or even of Thailand or Egypt is not an inviting one. What is not hypothetical, as John Knodel (1979) of the University of Michigan so cogently insists, is that such falls in fertility as have occurred in the badly off parts of the world, together with the marked increases in life expectation which have come about because of better health, are bringing into being large absolute, and increasingly relative, numbers of the aged, whose situation is entirely novel in their social structures and presumably unsuited to them. This realistic prospect is the less encouraging because of the great growth of cities in these societies, divorced from traditional social structure and traditional life.

The Achievement of the Fertility Decline

To return to the English case, to round off the discussion of the centrality of demographic experience, there are two particularly striking features of what has happened to us since the 1870s. First, it happened exceedingly fast, and secondly it was the consequence, though the entirely unintended consequence, of something else, something which was voluntary.

The fall in English fertility in the last hundred years has been sudden, even as historians reckon time, and virtually instantaneous as biologists do so. The later years of the last century are not far away as compared with the early sixteenth century, which must now be regarded as the beginning of accurate demographic record in our country. As for the voluntary character of this rapid change, all interferences with 'natural' fertility are reckoned to be like this to some degree. Certainly the actions of our Victorian, Edwardian, then Georgian predecessors in restraining their reproductive capacities went on at a time when fecundity was most probably rising. Until towards the end of the long period, up to our own day in fact, no really efficient contraceptive device was available. The evidence suggests that the commonest practices were withdrawal, abstinence, and the increasing use of the sheath, along with some deliberate abortion, and a little infanticide (Wrigley, 1969). The only important new evidence known to me to have appeared since Wrigley's study is that of the Mosher Archive, containing the results of a survey of the sexual and contraceptive behaviour of American professional women between 1892 and 1913. David and Sanderson (1978) in their analysis of this material insist that the practices in use, of which withdrawal represented less than half, were surprisingly successful, but decidedly demanding as to willpower. Coital frequency "was about 50 per cent lower than that observed in comparable population groups in the United States since the 1930s". It is not easy to see how representative the behaviour of this selected sample was for the rest of the American, or the English, population at the time, especially amongst the mass of the people but they must have behaved in a somewhat similar way.

Now these contraceptive practices are all highly self-conscious undertakings, and rather difficult as well. They require deliberate policy, especially on the part of the man. At this present time of highly effective, virtually automatic, chemical contraception it is already difficult to imagine how much voluntary determination went into the steady, monotonic decrease in births in England between the 1870s and the 1950s. In France the same concerted, yet supremely private, campaign went on from much earlier (Wrigley, 1970), at a time when methods may be supposed to have been even more dependent on decision. We are now well aware that these were not the earliest falls in fertility in demographic history, and that a voluntary element has been identified both in Europe and Japan (Smith, 1977); in the latter country child groups were deliberately planned by their parents to secure a particular sex composition as well as size, using infanticide. But never in the known records has fertility been deliberately controlled for so long and so drastically. Whatever we may think of the motives of these always patient, often frustrated, presumably frequently unsuccessful, but eminently determined Victorian and Edwardian couples, we are obliged to believe that they intended to reduce the number of their offspring.

The impression should not be given that up to the time of this decisive change in English procreative behaviour fertility had always been at very high levels, and families of children as big as those which are found in Africa or Indonesia today. We are now confident that in North-West Europe fertility was kept for much of our recorded history at consistently lower levels by lateness of marriage in women and by a relatively large proportion of people never marrying at all. This form of demographic regulation, which can be thought of as distinctively European, may well have been a reason why these areas were in a position to keep their populations to some extent above the level of subsistence and finally to escape from what we now define as under-development. However percipient Malthus may have been, it is a paradoxical fact that his famous principle, of growth in numbers always catching up with growth in resources, was being transcended at the very time and in the very country in which he announced it. Nevertheless the English continued to marry relatively late after they took to birth control on a considerable scale towards the end of the nineteenth century, and a proportion went on staying celibate. In the years leading up to the First World War, marriage age seems to have risen, and it has only been in the last half century or so that Western societies have taken to marrying early and almost universally, though still not to the extent of non-Western populations.

In one of the British Isles, in Ireland, this traditional European pattern of late marriage went to extremes in the earlier twentieth century. Irish fertility fell but not to the same extent as that of the English. There is an interesting question here about voluntariness in relation to individual and collective action, since in a sense traditional European modes of population regulation were voluntaristic: not to marry until or unless a viable opportunity presented itself could also be termed a willed decision.

It seems to me, however, that to prevent conception within marriage on such an unprecedented scale as was done in England in the later nineteenth century at the same time as traditional controls were still in use, at least to some degree, makes the case that the fall in fertility was an essentially willed affair even more persuasive. In more recent years when so much can be left to the pill and other highly reliable devices, the voluntariness of control is surely less conspicuous. Meanwhile, of course, all signs of traditional population regulation by postponed marriage seem to have disappeared. The recent tendency of proportions married to fall in the younger age group, accompanied as it is by the rise in procreative unions outside marriage, where procreation is nevertheless kept at the very lowest levels, cannot be thought of in the same way. The classic phase of voluntary contraceptive effort now lies in the past.

Some Problems

I have dwelt on the voluntary character of the fall in fertility in England in order to put two or three questions to you which are, I feel, of needling importance to our topic. Can it be supposed that all, many, or even any of the people who have acted in this purposeful way over the century which has elapsed since the 1870s also intended to bring about the ageing of the population of their country? Would it be reasonable to assume of the men and women of the 1980s who decide to have one, two or three children — and this will no doubt be most procreating couples — or even none at all, that they wish in this way to ensure that there shall continue to be a huge community of the elderly, relative to the rest of our population, a community which they themselves must inevitably join? Can such an outcome really be a part of the deliberate policy of those who applaud zero population growth at home, and who undertake to bring it about in countries which they describe as burdened with 'a population problem'?

We could pursue this rhetorical cross-examination, but with very little prospect of answers in the affirmative. In the historical case we have examined, it may be reasonable to suppose that the English persons who began limiting their families a century ago, and continued to do so for such a long time, were prepared to risk the *decline* of the population. But it would be quite unreasonable to hold them as in any way personally responsible for the *ageing* of the population, and even contemporary fathers and mothers, or couples who refrain from so becoming, must surely be for the most part held exempt. For what has been described is a signal example of the unintended consequences of decisions taken with entirely different purposes in mind, unintended but necessary, demographically necessary.

The medical men, the welfare officers and others who have had a part in lengthening life during the past century may have perhaps believed that they were engaged in expanding the population of the old in society in relation to the rest. If so, they were somewhat in error, not only because lengthening of life did not have this effect under the then prevailing demographic circumstances, but also because, as is now thought, it was the rise in the material standards of the mass of the population rather more than advances in medical or even in state welfare which improved the expectation of life, at least until the 1930s. What the doctors did was to help ensure that our population was kept from declining. Responsibility for our having collectively grown old must be firmly placed on those who deliberately controlled their child-bearing, and brought about the ageing of the population without meaning to do so. Demography of course is not the only source of conspicuous unintended consequences when individual in relation to collective behaviour is analysed. Those who now divorce themselves with such ease and in such numbers, an activity which is perhaps described as demography-related but which is certainly not properly demographic, are bringing on themselves the unintended consequence of diluting the filial kin ties whose strength and intensity will undoubtedly be important to them when they grow old.

Even to point these things out, of course, removes something of the quality of unintentionality from the actions of those who take cognisance of 'the way the demography works out'. Here then is my example intended to persuade you of the case for the centrality of demographic experience. It does, I hope, bear out the general claim which was made when we discussed demography in history and in literature: these are surely developments of the greatest significance to individuals and to collectivities. It is indeed difficult to think of weightier issues.

Such a story has the quality of tragic drama too, watching the actions of the myriads of persons who determinedly brought about an entirely unintended outcome for reasons concealed from them but now patent to the historian, the demographically informed historian. It certainly demonstrates, and in an urgent manner, how demography intervenes between the individual and the collectivity. For it requires us to decide how we can define 'social responsibility' when the unforeseen social consequences of individual actions can be so surprising and so serious.

Nevertheless a phrase like 'the centrality of demographic experience' is surely not likely to enter into an argument involving strict entailment. Although it seems obvious to me that the events which I have so lightly touched upon are correctly described as experience, experience undergone by a collectivity, the nation in the case of England, and experience on the part of English individuals too to some extent, it may still be correct to wonder whether the grammar of the word demography really goes like this. You may not wish to accept a simple distinction between demography as predominantly a matter of indices when applied to individuals, of experience when applied to collections of individuals. I should not complain.

Perhaps we ought not to be willing to leave so weighty a set of issues with no more serious or decisive comment. I confess that when I reflect on what may be the outcome of the rich, powerful, established, elderly nations of the world occupying the positions of strength, monopolizing the resources, keeping the younger populations out of their territory, away from the material and social goods, I cannot help but wonder. If you were to stand on the streets of Auckland, in the Northern Island of New Zealand, and watch the Tongans and the Cook Islanders at large amongst the indigenous population, you might wonder too. It is the same when you see the 'illegal immigrants' in the city of New York, and not very different as you contemplate what is going forward in the suburbs of London, the cities of the Midlands and the North.

Will it really come about that the populations from which these alien peoples spring will stay where they are, and as they are, until the whole population of the world becomes uniformly long lived, low in generative activity, and inordinately old, old as the definition we have set out here? "Let humanity prevail" can be the only plea to anyone who contemplates what could happen in a world undergoing this global demographic development. 'Centrality' we began by agreeing, is a suggestive rather than an exact way to approach the social reality which is outside us all but which is inside us too.

Since finally questions of morality slide so remorselessly into the discussion of issues which can only be understood with some knowledge of demography, we are surely justified in paying attention to all that may be conveyed by such a phrase as 'the centrality of demographic experience'.

References

Bertaux, D. (1979). Address given to a meeting on *Ageing and the Life Course*, Luxembourg in January 1979. Paris: Centre d'Etudes des Movements Sociaux.

Bogue, D.J. and Tsui A.O. (1979). *Zero World Population Growth*. Under review in *The Public Interest*, Spring.

David, P.A. and Sanderson, W.C. (1978). In *Proceedings of the Seventh International Economic History Conference*, Edinburgh, edited by M.W. Flinn. Edinburgh: Edinburgh University Press.

Demeny, P. (1979a). On the end of the population explosion. *Population and Development Review*, 5, 141–162.

Demeny, P. (1979b). Response to 'Reply to Paul Demeny'. *Population and Development Review*, 5, 479–494.

Easterlin, R.A. (1978). What will 1984 be like? Socioeconomic implications of recent twists in age structure. *Demography*, 13, 397–432.

Hammel, E.A. and Wachter, K.W. (1979). The chickens come home to roost. *Science*, 13, Autumn.

Knodel, J. (1979). Paper to the Cambridge Group, November.

Laslett, P. (1976). The wrong way through the telescope: a note on literary evidence in sociology and in historical sociology. *British Journal of Sociology*, 27, 319–342.

Laslett, P. (1977). *Family Life and Illicit Love in Earlier Generations*, Tables 5 and 6, p. 193. Cambridge: Cambridge University Press.

Laslett, P. (1979a). Illegitimate fertility and the matrimonial market. In *Marriage and Remarriage in the Populations of the Past*. Proceedings of an international conference on remarriage, Kristiansand, Norway, September 1979.

Laslett, P. (1979b). Family and collectivity. *Sociology and Social Research*, 63, 425–442.

Pressat, R. (1972). *Demographic Analysis*, Chapters 9 and 10. London: Edward Arnold.

Ryder, N. (1975). Notes on stationary populations. *Population Index*, 41, 3–28.

Smith, T.C. (1977). *Nakahara: Family Farming and Population in a Japanese Village, 1717–1830*. Stanford, California: Stanford University Press.

Tsui, A.O. and Bogue, D.J. (1978). Declining world fertility: trends, causes, implications. *Population Bulletin*, 33 (4), 1–54.

Wrigley, E.A. (1969). *Population and History*, p. 188 and References. London: Weidenfeld and Nicolson.

Wrigley, E.A. (1970). Family limitation in pre-industrial England. In *Population in Industrialization*, edited by M. Drake. New York: Barnes and Noble; London: Methuen.

Wrigley, E.A. (1978). Fertility strategy for the individual and group. In *Historical Studies of Changing Fertility*, edited by C. Tilly, Princeton: Princeton University Press.

Changing Patterns of Contraception

JOHN PEEL

Teesside Polytechnic, Middlesbrough, England

Contraception is the use of techniques which are designed to increase the interval between two pregnancies. Although amongst all human activities it is the most ubiquitous, it remains the most unpredictable in its outcome in any individual circumstance. And despite the fact that we can look back over almost a century of contraceptive history — a century which has seen such considerable progress in so many other spheres — it is remarkable how insubstantial the changes have been in the field of contraceptive practice.

The history of the general and systematic usage of contraception for the purpose of family limitation is almost precisely a hundred years old. Prior to the nineteenth century, fertility regulation was neither a public issue nor a personal preoccupation within the individual family. High birth-rates were counterbalanced by high death-rates and completed family size was thus kept within the then acceptable limits. These were the circumstances which provided Malthus with the evidence for his thesis that population and food supplies were kept in equilibrium only by the natural checks of pestilence, war and famine. During the nineteenth century however improved diet, the concern with personal hygiene and better methods of sanitation produced a dramatic fall in the death-rate, and this new imbalance in the Malthusian equation resulted in a closing of the gap between numbers of pregnancies and completed family size. A new and unique type of kinship structure resulted: the Victorian era was the first and last period in human history when the large, surviving family was the rule. Nor did it persist for more than a generation. By the late 1870s the birth-rate also began to decline to produce, in this century, the new norm of low birth-rates and low death-rates characteristic of all industralized societies.

The spectacular decline in the English birth-rate which began in 1877, and was referred to in detail by Professor Benjamin in an earlier paper, is one of the most remarkable features of world population statistics. 1877 was the year in which the legality of publishing contraceptive information was established in this country in the famous

41

Bradlaugh–Besant trial. This trial, involving two notable and respected public figures, attracted universal public interest and, by focusing attention on birth control as a feature of responsible parenthood, it provided an important catalyst in the process of family limitation. Contraceptive techniques, already used extensively outside the marriage relationship, now became acceptable adjuncts to planned family life. The diaphragm and the douche, previously used only by prostitutes and courtesans, now became indispensable aspects of motherhood whilst the condom, formerly a merely convenient receptacle for wild oats, was upgraded to an instrument of social change. Indeed, with the sole exception of the oral contraceptive, there is not a single method of contraception in use today which was not available in the last quarter of the nineteenth century. Even the intra-uterine device, in its infinite variety of shapes and forms, merited two full pages in the surgical catalogues of the 1880s.

It was on the basis of this array of contraceptive techniques — with *coitus interruptus*, then as now, playing a significant part in the process — that what has come to be termed the 'demographic transition' was achieved. The charting of the progress of this transition from decade to decade, by means of surveys designed to explore the various social class, occupational and geographical components of the process, is familiar ground to the student of population sociology. In each decade there has been shown to be an increase in the percentage of married couples using contraception at some time during their marriage accompanied by a corresponding increase in the proportion of couples using contraception from the outset of marriage. Table I summarizes this trend. These figures however represent merely quantitative changes in the adoption of a given range of techniques which, until the 1960s, were neither extended nor significantly improved. During most of the

Table I
Trends in contraceptive usage

Date of marriage	Percentage using contraception at some time during marriage
Before 1910	15
1910–1919	40
1920–1929	59
1930–1939	65
1940–1949	70
1950–1959	75
1960–1969	90
1970–1975	95

period *coitus interruptus* was the major method of contraception used, accounting for between 30 and 40 per cent of all using couples. The condom held a second position — again about 30 per cent of all using couples. The remaining 30 per cent of users comprised those using diaphragms and caps, the 'safe period', chemical contraceptives and other minor methods including sponges, Grafenberg rings and stem pessaries. There was, of course, considerable shifting between one method and another; in particular there was a tendency, revealed in successive surveys, for couples to change to a more effective method as desired family size was achieved or approached. Surveys revealed, too, certain social correlates for individual methods, age, social class, religion and length of education not only influencing choice of method but also the degree of success achieved by the use of a particular technique.

Informed interest in these matters in so far as it existed (and it was never a major preoccupation of the medical profession) tended to centre on the phenomenon of differential class fertility — the fact that the most inefficient contraceptors and the majority of non-contraceptors were found in the lowest socio-economic groups. It was in response to this problem that, from the early 1920s, groups of socially committed enthusiasts began to establish birth control clinics in London and other cities. In terms of their avowed aims — to bring birth control to the poor — these clinics were a failure. Their clientele consisted largely of middle-class women, most of whose contemporaries succeeded in finding adequate contraceptive techniques without resort to the clinics. Nor did these clinics significantly advance birth control technology. The two rival branches of the clinic movement — Marie Stopes on the one hand and the group later becoming known as the Family Planning Association — recommended competing vaginal barrier devices, the cap and the diaphragm respectively, and each condemned its opponents' technique as dangerous.

The birth control clinics never served more than ten per cent of women at reproductive risk and the vast majority of couples relied upon commercial sources, or upon non-appliance techniques, for their contraception.

It is clear, even from the crude percentage figures shown in Table I, that the disproportionate acceleration of the trend towards contraceptive usage which occurred in the 1960s must be a reflection of more fundamental and qualitative changes taking place in that decade. Indeed, the 1960s witnessed a revolution in attitudes to contraception and family planning in Britain. In that decade family planning became a predominant theme of public discussion in which newspapers, television, Parliament and the churches all played their part. Everybody, it seemed, had become birth control conscious to a degree.

Factors in Changed Attitudes to Family Planning

A number of factors clearly contributed to this changed outlook and the first of these was demographic. More people were marrying in the 1960s than ever before and they were doing so at earlier ages. More people were, in effect, becoming practically involved with the necessities of family planning. The unmarried, too, were coming face to face with opportunities for sexual experience previously unknown. The doubling of the numbers of young people in higher education, and therefore away from parental restraint, and the enormous earning potential of those who went to work in their 'teens were amongst factors which contributed to this greater sexual freedom. Its demographic outcome was a steep, and widely discussed, rise in the illegitimacy rate.

Secondly, an increasing concern with the world population explosion helped further to force family planning issues to the forefront of public discussion. Dr Timothy Black has described the 1960s as "the first international birth control decade" and it seems clear that the portrayal, in newspaper articles and on television, of the poverty, starvation and overcrowding in the Third World did more than the statistical predictions of the 1950s to bring home the reality of the problem of over-population. This international dimension had the effect of placing birth control studies on a more respectable basis than formerly, for whilst contraception, in its Western context, is concerned with the 'fun' end of the reproductive spectrum, thus providing an obvious target for the moralizing critics of permissiveness, on the world scale it came to be seen as a humanitarian pursuit of unprecedented importance.

The third, perhaps the most important, factor which led in the 1960s to our intense preoccupation with family planning was the addition — the first such addition for more than a century — to our traditional range of contraceptive techniques. Indeed, the influence of the pill, which was first introduced in this country in 1960, has far exceeded its importance as a technique of contraception. On the contrary, considered merely at a technical level it has had a disappointing performance; yet it was the pill which stimulated public discussion and debate and which provided the medical profession with what it saw as a legitimate professional concern in family planning. Even the debate on the health hazards of the pill had its positive side in calling attention to the

corresponding hazards involved in full-term pregnancy and the realization of these latter dangers became, in turn, an important issue in the
abortion debate which was an inevitable and logical outcome of the
discussions provoked by the pill. For once women are led to believe that
they can fully control their fertility by the use of an infallible method of
contraception, they are more likely to demand the right to terminate
unwanted pregnancies when these occur.

The relationship between contraception and abortion in the total
pattern of fertility control is complex and its clarification has only
become possible in the changed intellectual climate already mentioned.
Until ten years ago students of the demographic transition attributed the
late nineteenth century decline in the birth-rate solely to the increasing
use of contraception; the data summarized in Table I of this paper was
regarded as a sufficient explanation of the process. Neither in Banks'
classic work (Banks, 1954) nor in Glass's *Population Policies and
Movements in Europe* (1940) is there any explicit mention of induced
abortion as a contributing factor. Yet, in the 1930s this country had
already reached a condition of zero population growth — though the
term itself had not yet been adopted. To suggest that this could result
from a mere 65 per cent usage of traditional contraceptives is dubious
indeed. Even today, with 95 per cent of couples using contraception,
there is a need for 100 000 terminations annually.

The Arithmetic of Family Planning

The arithmetic of family planning in this country is clear and
unambiguous. According to the latest available data on contraceptive
usage (Family Planning Association, 1978), there are 11 million couples
in this country where the woman is of fertile age. Of these, approximately 1·1 million can be discounted because one or other of the couple
is infertile. At any one time a further 0·5 million couples are either
attempting to achieve a conception and in the case of an additional
600 000 couples one or other partner has been sterilized. This leaves 8·8
million couples with a problem of conception control and according to
the Family Planning Association the proportions amongst them using
different available options are as shown in the first column of Table II.

In the second column of Table II I have indicated, alongside each
contraceptive method, a failure rate — the most favourable failure rate
which I have seen published in the recent literature. This provides the
basis for the computation, in the final column of the table, of the mini-

Table II
Actual users of contraceptive methods in UK — October 1978

Method	Number of users (millions)	Failure rate (per HWY)	Expected annual accidental conceptions
Oral contraceptive	3·1	1·50	46 500
Condom	2·7	2·50	67 500
Withdrawal	0·7	10·00	70 000
IUD	0·6	3·50	21 000
Diaphragm	0·3	8·50	25 000
"Safe period"	0·2	15·00	30 000
Chemicals	0·1	10·00	10 000
Abstinence	0·7	—	—
Not using contraception	0·4	20·00	80 000
Total	8·8		350 000

HWY = hundred woman years.

mum number of accidental pregnancies which will occur due to contraceptive failure with each listed method. The total of these accidental conceptions amounts to 350 000 per year. To these must then be added the half million pregnancies occurring amongst that number of couples earlier excluded from the calculation because they were deliberately attempting to conceive. This provides a minimum national conception rate of 850 000. We know, however, that the number of live births in any recent year has never exceeded 800 000 and it seems logical to conclude, therefore, that the 50 000 legitimate conceptions which form our excess comprises that half of the annual 100 000 terminations which are performed on married women.

This very pragmatic exercise derives theoretical support from the work of Hulka (1969) who has shown that no reversible method of contraception currently available is adequate to allow fertility planning within the goals of family size now adopted in Western societies. Using a computerized model population he has demonstrated that, if one assumes a reproductive period of twenty years and a desired family size of three children, women marrying at the prevailing average age will have completed their families by their late twenties or early thirties with a further twelve to fifteen years of fertile life, and consequent exposure to the risk of unwanted pregnancy. If such women use methods of contraception which are 95 per cent effective then 30−35 per cent of these women may expect to have one unplanned pregnancy, 46−56 per cent may expect two or more unplanned pregnancies whilst only 13−18 per cent will not exceed their desired family size.

These statistical averages relate well, as I have shown, to community experience in an advanced industrial society. In societies less sophisticated in the use of contraception the need for induced abortion to counteract contraceptive failure will be more marked. No society has ever brought about a substantial reduction in its birth-rate by the use of contraception alone. It is of course open to any woman individually to attempt to defeat the statistics and to reduce the chances of an unwanted pregnancy by the use of a more effective method of contraception such as the pill. Unfortunately this involves a cost-benefit analysis in which contraceptive efficacy must be set against very positive health risks and in relation to the pill these increase dramatically as the woman approaches the age of forty. Tietze and his associates have constructed a model (Tietze, 1977) which compares the mortality risks associated with different methods of contraception with the mortality risks involved in unwanted pregnancy. They argue unequivocally that the use of traditional methods of contraception, e.g. the condom, combined with the use of early suction abortion for those failures that result, has the lowest level of mortality of any technique and is therefore the safest way at the present time for any woman to control her fertility. In making this recommendation, Tietze and his colleagues assume only a 90 per cent level of effectiveness for the condom and diaphragm, which is a level clearly surpassed by most users in this country.

The other possibility available to couples anxious to avoid the statistically inevitable unwanted pregnancy is surgical sterilization of one or other partner. However, although tubal ligation presents a smaller overall risk to life than any contraceptive method in younger women, an older woman is inviting a greater mortality risk by undertaking this option than by accepting early and repeated abortions. Vasectomy on the other hand is a procedure which, if carried out under local anaesthesia, carries virtually no mortality risk. It is a procedure which fulfils all the requirements which have been suggested for the ideal method of birth control: it is coitus-independent; it is virtually 100 per cent effective; it requires only one brief encounter between patient and doctor; it is less costly over a reproductive life-time than any other method of contraception, and it does not interfere with sexual performance. For all these reasons it has become a relatively popular choice in recent years for men whose desired family size has been attained. Although the absolute numbers of vasectomized men are small — probably no more than 200 000 — the rate of adoption of this technique during the ten years it has been generally available suggests that it may be the fastest growing form of contraception. Yet it is a technique with significant side-effects which has attracted considerable medical controversy, and its use is likely to be limited in the long run, in this country by the fact that it is difficult to obtain under the National Health Service, and in the United States because it is an important potential nexus for litigation in the prevailing pattern of medico-legal liability which bedevils clinical practice in that country.

Although a century of development and change in the field of contraception has not been marked by any technological advance which could be termed revolutionary, we have nevertheless arrived at a greater understanding of the role, and in particular the limitations, of contraception in the overall pattern of fertility control. Especially, the complex relationship between contraception and abortion is now regarded as positive and unavoidable (Potts *et al.*, 1977). A subsequent chapter in this volume reviews possible future methods of contraception, some of which may well avoid the limitations attaching to our existing range of techniques. If they do they will still have to be evaluated according to the cost — benefit equation of efficacy and health which is now recognized as a general feature of all medical provision. In the meantime we have a range of techniques which, despite their drawbacks, have been sufficiently effective to bring about a narrowing of the many social differentials formerly associated with variations in fertility. Socioeconomic status, occupation, length of education and religion still affect family building behaviour, but in each case there has been a convergence in recent years towards a national norm. On the world scale in relation to the population problems of developing countries it is likely that this avowedly eclectic approach to family planning will have more success than the mass IUD insertions and sterilization programmes attempted in the past. Again, in purely financial terms, the combination of traditional contraception with early abortion provides the most economical use of resources as well as the most efficient use of scarce medical manpower.

References

Banks, J.A. (1954). *Prosperity and Parenthood*. London: Routledge & Kegan Paul.

Family Planning Association (1978). Statement issued, 5th October 1978.

Glass, D.V. (1940). *Population Policies and Movements in Europe*. London: Routledge & Kegan Paul.

Hulka, J. (1969). A mathematical model study of contraceptive efficiency and unplanned pregnancies. *American Journal of Obstetrics and Gynecology*, **104**, 443.

Potts, M., Diggory, P. and Peel, J. (1977). *Abortion*, Chapter 13. London: Cambridge University Press.

Tietze, C. (1977). New estimates of mortality associated with fertility control. *Family Planning Perspectives*, **9**, 54−57.

Contraception in the Future

H.S.JACOBS

St Mary's Hospital Medical School, London, England

Prediction is perilous and the future infinite. This chapter is confined strictly to the foreseeable.

A comprehensive treatise is not appropriate, and there are already available some recent reviews (Short and Baird, 1976; Aitken, 1979; Connell, 1979). I shall select for discussion three departures that seem exciting to me, and end by suggesting that, in the particular case of contraception, the future remains firmly in the grip of the present.

The Chinese Connection

It is a rare privilege to be able to report a significant advance in male contraception. Gossypol is a phenolic compound that has been extracted from cotton plants and which impairs the fertility of male laboratory animals and of humans (Edwards, 1979). It has been used in China since 1972 and over 4000 men have been treated with it. It was discovered following the realization that in areas in which food is cooked in crude cotton seed oil, infertility in men is common.

In male rats the effect on spermatogenesis is dose related. Initially spermatids are affected, then as the dose is raised spermatocytes are damaged, and eventually the whole seminiferous tubule becomes depopulated. The interstitial cells are apparently not disturbed. In rats the effects on spermatogenesis are reversible, although they persist for four to five weeks after treatment has stopped. Apparently it takes up to 19 days to eliminate 98 per cent of the compound.

When humans are treated, infertility usually occurs after treatment for about two months with a dose of 20 mg per day by mouth. The maintenance dose is, however, lower. Evidently LH and testosterone secretion are not affected but the sperm count falls, abnormal spermatozoa appear in the ejaculate and eventually azoospermia develops. It may take three months for the sperm count to recover. The effect of Gossypol on the fertility of women has not yet been described.

Side effects do occur though they need to be characterized much more fully than hitherto. Muscular weakness is apparently common and changes in the cardiogram and the serum potassium have been recorded. These effects may be related to the subject's diet, since their prevalence apparently varies in different parts of China.

It is clear that the contraceptive action of Gossypol is an exciting discovery — the plant from which it is extracted is plentiful and, in contrast to the Mexican yam*, it grows widely and very readily. Indeed so numerous are the uses of cotton and cotton seed oil that it is intriguing to ask oneself whether contamination of food with this compound can explain the famous mystery of the falling American sperm count. It will be recalled that Smith and Steinberger (1977) reported that the frequency distribution of sperm counts in 'normal' American men has changed over the past thirty years, there being a marked shift to lower densities and smaller volumes. Indeed the mean total sperm count of normal American men has fallen from 350 000 000 in 1950 to 171 000 000 in 1977 (Smith and Steinberger, 1977). No-one knows the cause and indeed no-one knows if American men are less fertile now than they were thirty years ago. But cotton seed oil, given the current epidemic of coronary heart disease, is superficially attractive because of its very high content of polyunsaturated fatty acids, and apparently is available in certain foods at the moment. Thus, depending upon availability and price, it may constitute up to 10 per cent of soft margarine and of blended vegetable oils. In the United States, where it is legally required to reveal specifically what is in the 'foods' we eat, cotton seed oil can be seen to be in at least certain milk substitutes. Whichever way you look at it, Gossypol is going to be in the news. One only hopes it will be there as a contraceptive of the future rather than as a pollutant of the present.

The Sniff — a Swedish Solution

A more obviously endocrine advance has been the development of analogues of gonadotrophin releasing hormone for use as contraceptives. Ever since the isolation and characterization of the natural decapeptide LHRH, the chemists have been preparing analogues in the hope of obtaining a new method to control ovulation. Initially it was

---

* The source of the basic ingredient of the oral contraceptives in use today.

thought that to block ovulation an inactive analogue was needed which would bind on to LHRH receptors on pituicytes. These receptors would then not be activated, preventing the release of LH and FSH and so preventing follicular development and ovulation. At the same time superactive LHRH analogues were developed to provide a method for induction of ovulation in women with amenorrhoea. Paradoxically it was found that daily subcutaneous or intra-nasal treatment with a superactive analogue (D-ser (TBU)^6-EA^{10}-LRH) inhibited ovulation in women with regular menstrual cycles (Nillius *et al.*, 1978).

Berquist, Nillius and Wide (1979a) recently reported the results in 27 women of daily intra-nasal administration of this compound for three to six months (Fig. 1). Ovulation was inhibited in all but two of the 89 treatment months, and in the two failures (which occurred at the beginning of the study) there were apparently technical problems with the nasal spray. Twenty-one of the 27 women had slight menstrual-like anovular bleeds and the remainder were amenorrhoeic. There was however no post-treatment amenorrhoea.

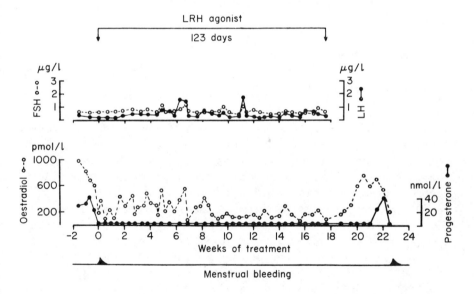

FIG. 1. Serum LH and FSH, and oestradiol and progesterone concentrations in a woman treated for 3 months with an intra-nasal preparation of a superactive LHRH analogue. Note the low levels and absence of cyclical fluctuations of LH and FSH concentration. Serum progesterone, low throughout the period of treatment (indicating the lack of ovulation), rapidly rose after treatment was stopped. From Berquist *et al.* (1979a) with permission of the authors and the editor of the *Lancet*.

The mechanism by which a superactive analogue inhibits ovulation is uncertain, but it seems that, after initial stimulation, LH and FSH secretion becomes inhibited (Fig. 2) (Nillius *et al.*, 1978). It is thought that exposure to pharmacological doses of a trophic stimulus 'down regulates' receptors and, in the present case, the pituitary becomes desensitized to stimulation by endogenous or indeed further exogenous gonadotrophin releasing hormone (Berquist *et al.*, 1979b).

Whatever the mechanism, the Swedish workers have clearly made a major advance in endocrine contraception. Perhaps the method will work in men too. I suspect, however, that the major problem will not prove to be endocrine, or even patient acceptability, but will be to do with its costs. LHRH is difficult to extract and so it (and its analogue) has to be chemically synthesized. A typical commercial preparation of the decapeptide used in diagnostic endocrinology costs almost £10 a dose. I do not know the cost of the analogue, but I doubt that it will be less. At present it is clearly a contraceptive of the future. Whether it will remain so or become one of those of the present will, I think, be decided in the boardroom rather than the laboratory or clinic.

Luteolysis — Sooner or Later

The great potential of a human luteolytic has been considered for several years and, of course, there was great hope that prostaglandins would fill that role. Taken early, a luteolytic could prevent implantation; taken later it might cause abortion. A luteolytic which inhibited the production of progesterone might even be used after the placenta has taken over steroidogenesis, either early in the pregnancy to induce abortion or later perhaps to induce labour.

The work of Csapo established that the human uterus will expel its contents after surgical removal of the corpus luteum during early pregnancy (Csapo and Pulkkinen, 1978). Moreover the abortion that results from luteoectomy can be prevented by replacement treatment with progesterone, but not by treatment with oestrogen (Fig. 2). The efficiency of surgical luteoectomy is closely related to the absolute level of plasma progesterone that follows the operation. If the operation is delayed until placental steroidogenesis makes a significant contribution to progesterone production, abortion does not result because progesterone levels do not fall sufficiently (Csapo and Pulkkinen, 1978).

Csapo has recently reported the use of isoxazole in rats (Csapo *et al.*, 1979). This drug inhibits the 3 beta steroid dehydrogenase enzyme and

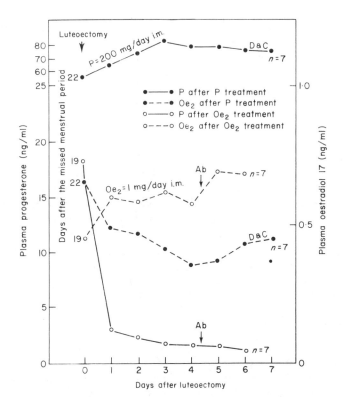

FIG. 2. The effects of treatment with progesterone or oestradiol on plasma steroid concentrations after luteoectomy of women during early pregnancy. Seven women (solid circles) who had injections or progesterone following the operation maintained plasma progesterone concentrations but had a fall of plasma oestradiol concentrations. These patients all required surgical termination of pregnancy.

Seven other women (open circles) had an injections of oestradiol after luteoectomy. These injections prevented the post-operative fall of oestradiol, but not the fall of progesterone. These seven women had spontaneous abortions. From Csapo and Pulkkinen (1978) with permission of the authors and the editors of *Obstetrical and Gynaecological Survey*.

so impairs progesterone secretion. Pregnancies are interrupted, the rate depending on the degree of suppression of progesterone production. An alternative approach has been to administer drugs which are peripheral antagonists of progesterone (Reel *et al.*, 1979). At present the use of peripheral antagonists of progesterone in man has not been reported. It has been known however for several years that inhibition of progesterone secretion by the corpus luteum could be achieved by suppression of the 3 beta steroid dehydrogenase enzyme, using synthetic progestogens. The results from *in vitro* studies of corpus luteum tissue obtained from women using mini pills, reviewed in detail by Fotherby (1977), indicate that inhibition of the 3 beta steroid dehydrogenase is the explanation for the subnormal endogenous progesterone secretion that typically occurs in 50 to 70 per cent of women using these preparations. The practicality of this approach to luteolysis is of course severely limited by the intrinsic progestogenic activity of synthetic progestogens. On the other hand, trilostane is an inhibitor of the 3 beta steroid dehydrogenase which has no intrinsic progestogenic activity. It has been used in humans to treat high blood pressure due to aldosterone excess and to treat Cushing's syndrome (Komanicky *et al.*, 1978). When given to women in the first trimester of pregnancy we have found that it suppresses progesterone secretion (Fig. 3) and, if the levels fall to below 5 ng/ml, abortion then results. Our early experience has been encouraging, but clearly more work needs to be done to establish optimum schedules.

The Future as Present

I have drawn attention to 3 potential advances in contraception and like to think they will become contraceptives of the future. But is there really a future for contraception? We all know we need some new approaches, that the rise in world population is out-stripping our reserves of food and energy etc., etc. But what of the politics and the economics of population control?

Firstly, how do you introduce a new contraceptive? There is a chilling account of the process by Elizabeth Connell (1979) in an excellent book on contraception to which reference has already been made. In brief the answer is, only with extreme difficulty. Current attitudes are against progress and it is a sad irony that the very people who campaign so forcefully against population growth are often those who consistently stress the negative aspects of pretty well any form of contraception short of abstinence. But that represents merely a psychological barrier to progress. There are more important bureaucratic and financial impediments. Consider first the cost. Djerassi (1976) calculates — and of all people he should know — that from first experiment to clinical use, the cost of a new contraceptive drug is of the order of $50 000 000. It is not a very inviting area for private enterprise and the record of non-capitalist investment in new contraceptives is dismal. Bureaucratic impediments to progress are also severe. The most important drug regu-

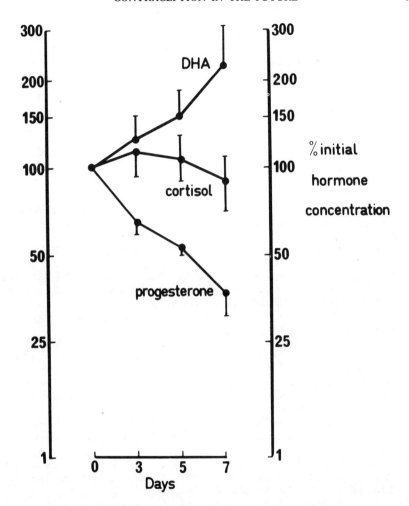

FIG. 3. Plasma progesterone, cortisol and dehydroepiandrosterone (DHA) concentrations in a group of pregnant women given trilostane during the first trimester of pregnancy. The results for each steriod concentration are expressed as a percentage of the mean pre-treatment concentration and they are plotted on a logarithmic scale. Plasma progesterone (product) concentrations fell to about 30 per cent of pre-treatment values in a week, during which time plasma DHA (precurser) concentrations rose to nearly 300 per cent of the pre-treatment level. There were no significant changes in plasma cortisol concentrations. From Jacobs, Wright and James, in preparation.

latory agency in the world is the Food and Drug Administration of the United States of America, and that agency is under constant pressure to assume a cautious and conservative posture (Connell, 1979). At present the process of introducing a new drug may take so long that by the time it is ready for the market the patent may have expired (Cromie, 1979). It has, for instance, already done so for norethisterone and norethynodrel.

In conclusion I fear that, despite the exciting compounds I have mentioned, the contraceptives of the foreseeable future will remain the contraceptives of the present.

References

Aitken, R.J. (1979). Contraceptive research and development. *British Medical Bulletin*, 35, 199–204.

Berquist, C. Nillius, S.J. and Wide, L. (1979a). Intra-nasal gonadotrophin-releasing hormone agonist as a contraceptive agent. *Lancet*, ii, 215–217.

Berquist, C. Nillius, S.J. and Wide, L. (1979b). Reduced gonadotrophin secretion in post-menopausal women during treatment with a stimulatory LRH analogue, *Journal of Clinical Endocrinology and Metabolism*, 49, 472–474.

Connell, E.B. (1979). Future methods of fertility regulation in clinics. *Obstetrics and Gynaecology*, 6, 171–184.

Cromie, B. (1979). The effect of British regulations. In *Medicine for the Year 2000*, edited by G. Teeling-Smith and N. Wells, pp. 75–83. London: Office of Health Economics.

Csapo, A.I. and Pulkkinen, M. (1978). Indispensability of the human corpus luteum, in the maintenance of early pregnancy: luteoectomy evidence. *Obstetrical and Gynaecological Survey*, 33, 69–81.

Csapo, A.I., Resch, B., Csapo, E.F. and Salau, G. (1979). Effects of antiprogesterone on pregnancy. 1. Midpregnancy. *American Journal of Obstetrics and Gynecology*, 133, 176–183.

Djerassi, C. (1976). The manufacture of steroidal contraceptives: technical versus political aspects. In *Contraceptives of the Future*, edited by R.V. Short and D.T. Baird, pp. 174–196. London: The Royal Society.

Edwards, R.G. (Editor) (1979). Gossypol, a new contraceptive for men. *Research in Reproduction*, 11 (3), 3.

Fotherby, K. (1977). Low doses of gestogens as fertility regulating agents. In *WHO Symposium on Advances in Fertility Regulation, Moscow USSR 1976*, edited by E. Diczfalusy, pp. 283–321. Copenhagen: Scriptor.

Komanicky, P., Spark, R.F. and Mellby, J.C. (1978). Treatment of Cushing's syndrome with trilostane (WIN 24,540), an inhibitor of adrenal steroid biosynthesis. *Journal of Clinical Endocrinology and Metabolism*, 47, 1042–1051.

Nillius, S.J., Berquist, C. and Wide, L. (1978). Inhibition of ovulation in women by chronic treatment with a stimulatory LRH analogue — a new approach to birth control? *Contraception*, 17, 537–545.

Reel, J.R., Humphrey, R.R., Shih, Y., Windsor, B., Sakowski, R., Greger, P.L. and Edgren, R.A. (1979). Competitive progesterone antagonists: receptor binding and biologic activity of testosterone and 19-nortestosterone derivatives. *Fertility and Sterility*, 31, 552–561.

Short, R.V. and Baird, D.T. (Editors) (1976). *Contraceptives of the Future*. London: The Royal Society.

Smith, K.D. and Steinberger, E. (1977). What is oligospermia? In *The Testis in Normal and Infertile Men*, edited by P. Troen and H.R. Nankin. New York: Raven Press.

Relative Risks in Fertility Control and Reproduction: Individual Choice and Medical Practice

SUE TEPER

Department of Community Health, University of Nottingham, Nottingham, England

Trends in Britain in the past twenty or thirty years towards almost universal use of birth control have been accompanied by a shift to 'medical' methods of contraception. 'Medical' in this context refers to steroidal techniques, the intra-uterine device and to abortion and sterilization. Individuals limit their fertility by using substances, devices and surgery obtained from or performed by the general practitioner, the family planning doctor or the gynaecologist.

With respect to fertility control, the medical role has altered drastically in the past half century, both in terms of clinical knowledge and also in relation to the 'problems' with which the doctor must deal. When Marie Stopes opened her birth control clinic in Holloway in 1921 she recommended almost exclusively the small cervical cap to be used with a suppository. Nearly one-quarter of the women who attended the clinic in its early years had been pregnant at least five times, frequently with barely noticeable intervals between delivery and subsequent conception. Some of the women had been pregnant 15 or more times (Stopes, 1925). In Glasgow, in the nineteen twenties and thirties, Dugald Baird saw the effects of rapid, uncontrolled and excessive child-bearing — and the attitudes of the medical profession towards it. In Aberdeen he offered therapeutic abortion and sterilization to grand multiparae. At that time, both procedures carried significant risks of morbidity and mortality. Twenty years ago medical practitioners were able to prescribe oral contraception without any concern about cardio-vascular disease. There were, however, some general fears about the effects of steroids on any future progeny, and some very specific fears about their effect on morality! Young, unmarried women had begun to appear as family planning attenders.

In recent years, together with developments in contraceptive technology there has come a greater awareness and knowledge of the risks associated with particular mechanisms for controlling fertility. Work published by Vessey and his colleagues, and the results of a study carried out under the auspices of the Royal College of General Practitioners, demonstrate that women who have used the pill are subject to excess death rates from circulatory diseases when compared with women who have never taken the pill (Vessey, *et al.*, 1977; Royal College of General Practitioners, 1977). It is known that there are complications arising from IUD use — in particular, should the device fail and the user become pregnant, the risk of an extra-uterine pregnancy is increased by a significant factor (Seward *et al.*, 1972; Vessey *et al.*, 1974; Perlmutter, 1978). A recent study by the World Health Organisation has shown that even when abortion is induced in excellent facilities there is an increased risk of spontaneous abortion of premature delivery in the next pregnancy (World Health Organisation, 1979a).

Knowledge about the control of reproduction continues to increase by leaps and bounds, but there is not — as yet — a *perfect* contraceptive. The proliferation and growing sophistication of fertility control methods means that the doctor is expected to possess a truly enormous technical knowledge in order to 'prescribe' contraception. That knowledge and its use are — for the most part — only a small segment of his or her medical practice.

The other side of the coin is represented by the needs of those people who wish to control their fertility. What do individuals demand of their fertility control? First, and most basic of all, is that the method selected be acceptable to the individual who plans to use it. Secondly, but of almost equal importance, it must give adequate protection against unwanted pregnancy. Thirdly, the method chosen should leave future fecundity unimpaired.

Fourthly and finally, contraception must carry minimal risks of morbidity and mortality. 'Risk' in a statistical sense must be differentiated from 'risk' as seen by the individual. At an individual level, what matters to each woman is whether she *herself* will die from a cerebral haemorrhage as a result of using oral contraception, in contrast to the statistician's way of thinking who knows that the numbers who do so are very low. The situation can be likened to the very low risk of a bomb exploding aboard an aircraft flight. To the individual woman it is not the small number of bombs that matters — it is whether one actually goes off while she is on board the aircraft; and when she is, for example, using oral contraception there is a bomb 'on board' every day.

This introduction has attempted to demonstrate that an important interface exists between:

(1) the hazards of fertility control techniques, as known to the

medical profession; and

(2) the needs and preferences of the individual who wishes to limit his or her fertility*.

In abstract terms, the provision of services for family limitation involves a strategy which minimizes risks to health and life, and maximizes individual success and satisfaction with both reproduction and its control. For the individual these factors change over time — and thus the strategy must be flexible. The power of the medical profession in resolving the problems of the interface, and in translating strategy into reality, is vast. In this paper we are concerned with the first part of the interface — the hazards of fertility control.

The next section deals with the various aspects of fertility control. Acceptability and efficacy are discussed, followed by consideration of the effects on subsequent fertility for the major methods. The effect of failed contraception on the foetus is also included. A review of the 'hazards' is then presented, first for birth control methods, and then for abortion, sterilization and finally childbirth. Sets of risk factors are presented. A discussion section completes the chapter.

Aspects of Fertility Control

BIRTH CONTROL

Acceptability

In theory at least, a variety of factors may be taken as 'measures' of acceptability for specific contraceptive techniques. In practice, from the various studies on the epidemiology of reproduction the only possible measure which can actually be used is discontinuation of one method in association with initiation of an alternative method. However, within a group of women who do change methods there would be a substantial proportion who had done so because the side-effects of a particular method had made it intolerable to them. In the introduction, and in the broader context of this paper, *acceptability* is used at a very personal level. There are a large number of what are essentially psychosexual factors which affect the ability and motivation of an individual or couple in relation to their contraceptive activity. The definition and scope of these factors is well beyond the scope of this paper.

---

* The issue of restricting cost is also pertinent. For reasons of economy of space it is not covered here.

Protection Against Unwanted Pregnancy

Traditionally, in the evaluation of contraceptive methods a distinction is drawn between *theoretical effectiveness* and *use-effectiveness*. Theoretical effectiveness refers to "the antifertility action of a method or production under ideal conditions" (Tietze and Lewit, 1968; see also MacLeod and Tietze, 1964). It represents the performance of a method under laboratory conditions; and it is therefore, to all intents and purposes, an abstract concept. For a method such as oral contraception, theoretical effectiveness may well approach 100 per cent. Use-effectiveness represents a measurement of the success with which a specified population uses a particular method (Tietze, 1959). It is with use-effectiveness that this section of the chapter is concerned.

Pregnancy rates can be calculated using Pearl's formula, which relates unwanted pregnancies to the aggregate of all exposure (in terms of months). The result is expressed as a rate per 100 woman-years of use. To a large extent this approach has been replaced by the use of the life table, a more sensitive and flexible tool. Cumulative pregnancy rates are calculated in *gross* terms in a *single-decrement* table. *Net* rates appear in multiple-decrement tables in which allowances are made for the various reasons for method discontinuation (Potter, 1966).

Most data on the effectiveness of contraception come from clinical studies of specific methods. These may be supported by the manufacturer of the product, they may be undertaken by clinicians in the course of their work, or they may be completed by or in collaboration with one of the international agencies — such as the World Health Organisation. The major disadvantages of these sources are (1) that, in a *demographic* sense, *total* populations are not covered (see below), and (2) that frequently the format of the studies, their results and publications relating to them make comparisons between studies — and therefore between methods — dubious, difficult or impossible. There is, fortunately, one further source of data available. This source provides base-line information on the risks of unwanted pregnancy by method. It is a particularly simple set of data, and it enables us to examine the problems of measurement and interpretation which occur in this sphere.

In 1970 and 1971 information was collected on women's reproductive histories in a national fertility survey in the United States. Those interviewed were selected on the basis of a national probability sample. Questions on contraceptive failure were included in the study (though the data suffer from the limitation that the information was collected on a retrospective basis). The methodology used is expertly described by Ryder (1973). In the enquiry, and in the presentation of the results, contraceptive intent was partitioned into whether conception was inten-

Table I

Percentage of contraceptors who fail to delay a wanted pregnancy or to prevent an unwanted pregnancy in the first year of exposure to risk of unintended conception, by method (United States National Fertility Study, 1970)

Method	Intention		
	Delay	Prevention	Both categories
Pill	7	4	6
IUD	15	5	8
Sheath	21	10	17
Diaphragm	25	17	23
Foam	36	22	31
Rhythm	38	21	33
(n_i)	(3719)	(2233)	(5952)

Source: Ryder, 1973.

tional or accidental, and if accidental, whether the intent prior to conception was to *delay* the next conception or to *prevent* it altogether.

Table I shows data on contraceptors who failed to delay a wanted (wanted later) pregnancy or to prevent an unwanted pregnancy in a single year of exposure to the risk of unintended conception. The figures are given separately for the various methods. The rates are of a life table type. The ranking for the methods (for prevention or delay) in decreasing order of effectiveness is the pill, the intra-uterine device (IUD) and sheath; followed by the diaphragm, foam and rhythm. Considering delay or prevention separately leaves the ranking of methods unchanged. As might be expected, success at 'prevention' is greater than success at 'delay' for each method — sometimes by a considerable factor. The difference for the IUD — 15 per cent for delay compared with five per cent for prevention — at first seems surprising. To understand this three-fold difference it is necessary to look in more detail at the structure and meaning of data on contraceptive behaviour.

A failure rate with a particular contraceptive is not an estimate of the intrinsic anticonceptional properties of the method itself. Such a rate obviously reflects such a property, but it also reflects the characteristics of the users themselves. A couple may find a method unacceptable and discontinue, and if an alternative is not instituted immediately an unwanted pregnancy may occur. In Ryder's work this type of failure is allocated to the initial contraceptive method. Although this moves measurement firmly away from theoretical effectiveness, it does mean that measurement reflects actual human behaviour.

In the data of Table I particular characteristics of the users which affect the resultant figures have been subsumed. Age, previous contraceptive experience and previous obstetric history all affect success with a method. In addition, particular methods may be associated with lower success rates simply because they are used by people more concerned with delay than prevention. This certainly applies to the IUD, which in addition can have a fairly high discontinuation rate. These factors are likely to account for the differences in the columns of Table I.

From within the 1970 data set itself and also from a later study (Vaughan *et al.*, 1977), a secular trend has become evident in terms of an increase in success at preventing unwanted pregnancy (the two studies are not exactly comparable). This improvement reflects a shift towards better methods (that is, greater use of methods with an intrinsically high rate of effectiveness — such as the pill) plus method-specific improvements (that is, better care in the use, or more consistent use, of any of the methods). Although such shifts can be expected, they will on the whole leave *crude* factors of *relative* risk *between* the methods more or less unchanged.

The data of the National Fertility Study can be used to summarize some of the basic features of contraceptive use which need to be considered when interpreting use-effectiveness data, whatever their source:

1. Use-effectiveness in a total population is always less, and sometimes very much less, than theoretical effectiveness. It will also generally be lower than that observed in clinical studies (see below).
2. Contraceptive methods — *as used* — can be clearly ranked by effectiveness at delaying or preventing unwanted pregnancy.
3. The reason for use — delay or prevention — influences success with a method.
4. Success at contraception is "the *joint consequence* of method characteristics and user characteristics" (Ryder, 1973).

These US data can be used for background information against which material collected from clinical situations can be compared. Current clinical material can be expected to yield better results for two reasons. First, the 1970 data are known to be somewhat out of date. For example, Vaughan's work for the US for 1970–73 gives figures of 2·9 (prevention), 5·6 (delay) and 4·2 (both categories) for the IUD — compared with the 5, 15 and 8 per cent for 1970–71 from Table I (Vaughan *et al.*, 1977; US Department of Health, Education and Welfare, 1979). Secondly, the range of personal characteristics and behaviour in the population of a clinical study may be less wide-ranging than in a national population as a whole.

As an illustration of material from clinical sources data published on the IUD this year are included (Table II). Any real comparison between these results involves using details of the study designs and the study populations. One-year pregnancy rates range from 0·6 to 2·0 per 100 woman-years, depending on the type of device. They are, therefore, less than those for a whole population (differences between various forms of any single method are dealt with in succeeding sections of this chapter). In an interesting two-year study of early *post-partum* insertion of the Multi-load 250 in Birmingham four pregnancies occurred amongst 162 insertions, all in the first three months after insertion (Emens, *et al.*, 1978). Unfortunately the published material does not allow the conversion of this information into rates — life table, Pearl or others — which are comparable with the other studies. This kind of lack of comparability is a frequent, and disappointing, feature of material deriving from clinical situations.

Future Fecundity

Data on the return of fertility after discontinuation of the various contraceptive methods in order to conceive are available from the Oxford Family Planning Association contraceptive study (Vessey *et al.*, 1978). The data indicate that the return of fertility is delayed longer in oral contraceptive users in comparison with women who have discontinued the use of other methods; and that this applies to both parous and nulligravid women. Some of the data from this study are shown in Table III. The salient features of the results are that the difference between oral contraception and other methods disappears after 30 months for parous women and 42 months for women who had never had a pregnancy; the results are independent of the length of pill use. Most of the

Table II
One-year pregnancy rates per 100 women; IUDs by selected device: 1979 reports

Device	No. of insertions	Woman-months of use	Pregnancy rate per 100 women
Unmedicated Lippes Loop D	894	9275	2·0
Medicated TCu-220C	889	9952	0·6
Nova T	907	8790	0·7

Sources: TCu-220C and Lippes Loop D from World Health Organisation 1979b. Nova T from Luukkainen *et al.*, 1979.

Table III
Fertility of women after they stopped using different methods of contraception in order to conceive

Women who stopped using:	Gravidity status		% of women remaining undelivered at various intervals after discontinuing contraception (in months)					
			12	18	24	30	36	42
Oral contraception	Nulligravid	1174	70.1+1.3(737)	32.8±1.4(318)	20.8±1.2(176)	16.1±1.2(123)	12.8±1.1(85)	10.7±1.1(57)
Diaphragm		394	46.4±2.3(166)	23.4±2.1(80)	16.7±1.9(53)	13.7±1.8(37)	10.6±1.7(23)	9.5±1.6(16)
IUD		8	31.5	–(2)	–(1)	–(0)	–	–
Other		377	48.9±2.4(159)	21.7±2.1(65)	14.1±1.9(38)	12.8±1.8(25)	10.3±1.8(14)	9.5±1.8(11)
Oral contraception	Parous	1060	59.9±1.5(509)	20.0±1.3(144)	10.4±1.1(62)	6.9±0.9(34)	4.3±0.8(17)	3.5±0.8(10)
Diaphragm		661	35.2±1.7(198)	11.8±1.2(60)	7.1±1.1(31)	5.2±1.0(21)	3.2±0.8(12)	– (8)
IUD		258	48.5±3.2(93)	17.0±2.5(27)	8.5±2.1(10)	– (6)	– (1)	– (1)
Other		424	38.5±1.2(412)	13.5±1.0(122)	8.1±0.8(58)	5.8±0.8(36)	3.8±0.7(20)	3.4±0.6(14)

Results are percentages (± s.e.) of women remaining undelivered of stillbirth or live birth at intervals after stopping contraception. Numbers of women remaining undelivered and under observation are shown in parentheses.
Source: Vessey et al., 1978.

women were 25 or over at the time of recruitment, and the population, therefore, contains few women who began the use of oral contraception during their teenage years.

The Oxford study contains a relatively small number of women using the IUD — 258 multiparous women and only eight never-pregnant women. More extensive information on the IUD from other sources confirms, however, that no deleterious effect on fertility can be expected (Segal and Tietze, 1971; Tietze and Lewit, 1970). This does not apply if the user has developed pelvic inflammatory disease (see p. 76). There is some disturbing evidence from Taiwan, which suggests that the longer a woman uses an IUD the less are her chances of conception after discontinuation relative to non-users of the same age. Jain and Moots (1977) demonstrated that the proportion of women aged 35 and over with three years IUD use who failed to conceive was three times the rate for matched women with only one year of use.

Since accidental pregnancy can occur during pill use or with an IUD *in situ*, it is appropriate to consider the outcome of these pregnancies and to determine whether the children born have an increased risk of congenital abnormalities. Approximately 50 per cent of uterine pregnancies conceived with the IUD in place end in spontaneous abortion if the device is left (Alvior, 1973; Shine and Thompson, 1974; Vessey *et al.*, 1974). This is 4 to 8 times the risk for women without a device (Shine and Thompson, 1974). Removing the device during pregnancy reduces the risk of miscarriage by half or more (Alvior, 1973; Snowden *et al.*, 1977). Leaving the device, or having to leave the device, may increase the risk of premature delivery or stillbirth (Alvior, 1973; Shine and Thompson, 1974). One worker has reported that four times as many premature births occurred if Copper Ts were left in place as when they were removed (Tatum, *et al.*, 1976). Finally, there is no evidence to suggest that an infant born in these circumstances has an increased chance of suffering from any congenital anomaly (Snowden, *et al.*, 1977; Perlmutter, 1978). The likelihood of an ectopic pregnancy with an IUD *in situ* is discussed later in this paper (see p. 76).

In the Royal College of General Practitioners' contraceptive study, 136 women who conceived accidentally whilst using oral contraception continued (inadvertently) to take the pill. Of the pregnancies 102 went to term; and there were nine babies with abnormalities of which two were congenital. None of the abnormalities could be directly attributed to hormone ingestion during the early part of the pregnancy. The pattern of pregnancy outcome following discontinuation of oral contraception is relatively similar to that of the controls. This supports the earlier findings of the study (Royal College of General Practitioners,

1974). The report concludes that "there is now strong evidence that oral contraceptive usage has no material effect on subsequent births. However, it is difficult to exclude a very small risk" (Royal College of General Practitioners, 1976).

Morbidity and Mortality

Evidence on the hazards ascribed to any one particular contraceptive method is often confusing and frequently the findings of one worker conflict with those of another. Animal-based studies may or may not be generalizable to man. Clinical trials may have been carried out with subjects who are white, married urban residents of an American city, who are nulliparous and live in the south of England or who are parous villagers in rural Thailand. Subjects, study designs and contraceptive method all vary, and the purpose of this section is to draw some conclusions from the work undertaken so far.

A review of risks associated with fertility control is of necessity selective. Many sources have been used, including specialized review papers. There was a clear choice between presenting risks by methods or methods by risks, both of which would have been lengthy. We, therefore decided to present only the salient features. Given the predominance of female methods amongst those with known health hazards, it is hardly surprising that discussion of the techniques used by women forms the core of this chapter. We have concentrated on methods used in the United Kingdom, although evidence on risks has been drawn from international sources. Accordingly menstrual regulation, post-coital contraception and injectable steroids have not been included since they are not widely used in this country. Because of the importance of fertility and its control to developing societies, the Third World situation has been included briefly in the discussion at the end of the chapter.

As a starting point the following simple classification is useful. Health risks associated with contraception can be grouped as follows:
Side-effects
Longer-term systemic effects (including, for example, the development of neoplasia)
Mortality

Side-effects with oral contraception include headache, weight gain, fluid retention, depression, change in libido, and so forth (Hunton, 1976). A change of brand may improve the situation; and in general low dose preparations are associated with a lower incidence of side effects (Ingemanson *et al.*, 1976; McEwan, 1977). With a progestogen-only regimen disturbances of the menstrual pattern are frequent (Soutoul *et al.*, 1976; Fotherby, 1977).

With the IUD the most frequent complaints are heavy bleeding and pain. Menstrual flow may be increased, both in terms of volume and duration, and between-cycle spotting may occur (Guillebaud *et al.*, 1976). Copper-clad devices increase bleeding, but to a lesser extent than non-medicated devices (Morehead *et al.*, 1975; Guillebaud, *et al.*, 1976). Progestogen-releasing devices reduce the flow (Nilsson, 1977). Perforation and expulsion may occur on insertion or subsequently. Tatum has reviewed the risks of perforation (Tatum, 1977) and Lippes has remarked "IUDs do not perforate. For this to happen we need a practitioner" (Lippes, 1978). One-year event rates for expulsion range from 2·2 with the TCu-200 (Timonen and Luukkainen, 1974) to 15·5 with the Cu-7 (Jain and Sivin, 1977). Different estimates can be obtained from the various reports for the same device. Endocarditis and septicaemia have been reported soon after insertion or removal (Guillebaud, 1978).

In relation to *longer term effects* we know that the use of oral contraception is associated with a small but significant rise in blood pressure. This is reversible on withdrawal of the drug (Fisch and Frank, 1977). A tiny proportion of women develop overt hypertension (Kaulhausen and Klingsiek, 1976). There is as yet no screening procedure for identifying those women amongst pill-takers who are at risk of developing serious cardiovascular disease, but undoubtedly in some women long-term and undetected pathological changes occur. Oral contraceptives have been variously implicated in the development of neoplasms — or in some cases in providing protection against them — in relation to such sites as breast, cervix and liver, which we discuss later (a review is available in Population Reports, 1977). A clear link has been established between gall bladder disease and oral contraception (Royal College of General Practitioners, 1974). The results of one study have suggested that younger women likely to develop gall bladder disease tend to do so within 6 – 12 months of starting the pill; an age-standardized risk factor of 2 has been postulated in comparison with non-users (Boston Collaborative Drug Surveillance Program, 1973).

Amongst IUD users the most serious long term effect is the development of pelvic inflammatory disease (PID). This can occur in one of many forms, several of which have the potential to produce sterility. As we mentioned in the introduction, should pregnancy occur with a device *in situ* then the risk that the pregnancy will be ectopic is significant.

Reports of excess *mortality* among pill users can be found in relation to disease of the circulatory system. There were a small number of deaths from septic abortion among women with IUDs — these occurred mainly in the United States in the early 1970s, and the particular device in question was the Dalkon shield (Cates *et al.*, 1976).

The *longer* term effects outlined above (with the exception of gall bladder disease) and mortality from cardiovascular disease are discussed below. For this chapter we intend to attempt a synthesis of the available evidence in the four following — and major — areas:

Neoplasia and the pill;
Pelvic inflammatory disease and the IUD;
Ectopic pregnancy and the IUD;
Cardiovascular disease and the pill.

Neoplasia

Given the widespread interest in cancers, it is not surprising that possible links between the development of neoplasms — both benign and malignant — and oral contraception have attracted a substantial amount of interest. With some neoplasms, for example those of the breast, there is evidence that *endogenous* hormones affect development, and it might be reasonable to postulate some link with pill use. Irrespective of site, reports of neoplasia in women taking hormones, whether for therapeutic purposes or as a contraceptive agent, come from many sources. The results, with one or two exceptions, are not particularly striking. Part of the reason for this may be that the link between neoplasia of particular sites and oral contraception is not substantial; or that any clear links have yet to become observable when cohorts with major and long-term exposure to the pill age and develop the diseases. However, there are factors in the epidemiology of neoplasia which make it particularly difficult to identify and establish what links there may be. This arises because most of the tumours are rare, their incidence does not change rapidly over time, the aetiology of an individual disease frequently remains unknown or uncertain, and the diagnosis and classification of specific neoplasms lack consistency.

Breast. Most of the studies which have been completed show no link, either positive or negative, between the use of oral contraception and breast cancer. One study in California found more oral users than expected in some sub-groups of breast cancer patients (Fasal and Paffenbarger, 1975). This was not supported in a British study which covered some of the same population/user groups (Vessey, *et al.*, 1975).

Most of the debate about pill use and breast lesions surrounds *benign* breast disease — usually the incidence of fibroadenoma or fibrocystic disease. The majority of studies have demonstrated that pill users are less likely than others to develop benign breast disease. The protective effect takes on statistical significance over two or more years of use (Population Reports, 1977), and it is more pronounced in long-term users (British Medical Journal, 1976). The protective effect appears to apply less to fibroadenomata which tend to occur in younger women and do not appear to be precursors of malignant disease, than to fibrocystic diseases. Cystic disease tends to occur in middle aged women, it occurs more frequently than the adenomas, and there is a link between some types of fibrocystic disease and cancer (Monson et al., 1976).

It is well established that women who develop benign breast lesions are more likely to become breast cancer patients than other women (Donnelly et al., 1975). The link from benign disease to carcinoma is, however, not straightforward. In an epidemiological sense the two diseases are different (Ory et al., 1976). Oral contraception may well turn out to protect against those forms of cystic breast disease which do not lead to subsequent malignant disease. There is some evidence to this effect, i.e. that the type of cystic disease which is little, if at all, likely to lead to breast cancer is the one against which the pill protects (Livolsi et al., 1978). The most recent evidence on the *magnitude* of the protective effect puts it at some 80 per cent for any use of oral contraception (Vessey et al., 1979).

Finally, it should be noted that when patients with breast cancer have been matched according to use or non-use of oral contraception, oral users have been found to have less axillary disease than non-users. Use of oral contraception may, therefore, exert a retarding effect on the spread of breast cancer (Briggs and Briggs, 1978).

Cervix. Evidence on the link between cervical neoplasia and the pill has so far been inconclusive — some studies have found a positive association, others have not. The area is complicated by a number of factors. Firstly, mystery continues to surround the natural history of cancer of the cervix. Secondly, although an associative, though not causal, link has been established between early first intercourse, multiple partners and cervical disease, the use of the pill confounds the issue. Thirdly, in most cases the development of cervical disease is a long process in terms of time. And finally, there is lack of consistency in the diagnosis and classification of cervical lesions.

Two case-control studies in north America on white populations have found no association between the use of oral contraceptives and biopsy-proven cervical neoplasia (Thomas, 1972; Worth and Boyes, 1972). A further study on a black American population, which controlled for age at first intercourse, also found no association (Boyce *et al.*, 1977). A fourth case-control study — also on a black American population — found a strong positive association between carcinoma *in situ* and pill use (Ory *et al.*, 1977). The link was dependent on length of use, and women who had used the pill for three or more years had a risk factor five times that of the controls. It should, however, be noted that in all four studies *mean* duration of pill use was short — less than three years in all cases.

The findings from cohort studies have also been inconclusive: half have found some association and half have not (Vessey, 1979). Results from the Oxford Family Planning Association study show similar rates of proven cervical neoplasia in pill users and IUD users, but drastically lower rates in those who entered the study using the diaphragm (see Table IV) (Vessey, 1979). Barrier methods obviously offer considerable protection against the disease.

Work on cervical neoplasia and oral contraception has been concentrated in the United States, Britain and Canada. Rates of cancer of the cervix are much higher in other parts of the world and there is an urgent need for sound epidemiological studies to be established in some of these countries (Table V). Although it is disconcerting to find conflicting evidence in the two black American studies, the fact that black Americans have different patterns of age at first birth, and age at first intercourse (Presser, 1971), may mean that the work of Ory and his colleagues will be confirmed at a later date in the white population of America.

Uterine body. An increased incidence of endometrial carcinoma was suspected in women using oral contraception in its sequential form (Cohen and Deppe, 1977). Sequentials, however, were taken by only a small proportion of users, and the products have now been withdrawn. The question of risks associated with the use of oestrogens at the meno-

Table IV

Oxford Family Planning Association Study. Incidence rates for biopsy proven cervical neoplasia (dysplasia, carcinoma in situ, *or invasive carcinoma) per 1000 woman-years of observation.*

Method of contraception	Rate per 1000 woman-years	(n_i)
Pill	0·95	(47)
IUD	0·87	(14)
Cap	0·17	(4)

Source: Vessey, 1979.

Table V

Reported annual incidence of cancer of the uterine cervix, rate per 100 000 women, 1960 or later

Country	Saskatchewan, Canada	Kingston and St Andrews, Jamaica	Denmark	German Democratic Republic	Scotland
Rate per 100 000 women	11·4	29·5	37·9	42·1	13·6

Source: Population Reports, 1977.

pause remains controversial. This is an area outside the scope of this paper, but a review is available (Population Reports, 1977). In a study undertaken by the Royal College of General Practitioners it was found that pill users were less likely to develop uterine fibroids — benign uterine tumours — than other women (Royal College of General Practitioners, 1974). This finding was not supported in another British study, and it may simply be a function of selection factors (Vessey *et al.*, 1976). Oral contraception following treatment for hydatidiform mole may be related to the subsequent development of a trophoblastic — and malignant — tumour (Stone *et al.*, 1976).

Ovary. There is no evidence to suggest that pill taking is associated with any increase in the incidence of ovarian tumours. Some studies show a protective effect against benign, functional ovarian cysts (these are not true neoplasms) (Ory, 1974). From Finland we have data which show a markedly higher than normal incidence of such cysts in women taking progestogen-only therapy — this may reflect anovulatory cycles with hormonal changes (Ylikorkala, 1977). In the interpretation of data relating to the ovary however, a careful distinction is not always made in the studies between functional cysts and neoplasms.

Liver. Reports on some 200 or so cases of women who developed liver tumours while on the pill appeared in the medical journals between 1973 and 1977. Before this period such tumours had occurred only very rarely in young women. The subject was important enough to merit an editorial in the British Medical Journal of 1977 (British Medical Journal, 1977). The majority of tumours were benign in structure: they were either focal nodular hyperplasias or hepatocellular adenomas. Some 13, however, were (or had perhaps progressed to) hepatocellular carcinomas; that is, they were malignant. Hyperplasias were generally diagnosed at surgery for some other problem. These lesions seldom lead to complications. Adenomas may rupture, and since they tend to be highly vascular, this can be fatal (Nissen *et al.*, 1977). The risk of developing a tumour increases with duration of pill use. In one series, mean duration of oral contraceptive use was in excess of six years (Edmondson *et al.*, 1976). There is still uncertainty as to whether *both* types of liver neoplasms are related to oral contraceptive use. Mestranol, the main synthetic oestrogen used in the period prior to 1977 has been implicated, but this may be purely artefactual (Edmondson *et al.*, 1976; Keifer and Scott, 1977).

The risk of pill users compared to controls is shown in Table VI. In relation to neoplasms of the breast there is a clear protective effect against some *benign* tumours. This protection probably only applies to those forms of the disease which are unlikely to precede malignancy. A link with cancer of the breast — in either direction — has still to be established. There may be an increased association between pill use and carcinoma *in situ* of the cervix. The work of Ory and his colleagues has yet to be confirmed; his present estimate of the risk factor is 5. Because this has not been generally supported it has been marked with a question mark in Table VI. The findings in relation to the corpus uteri are uncertain. Pill users may be less likely to develop fibroids; however, sub-fertile women who are more likely to develop them may well be less likely to use oral contraception. There seems to be a link between evacuation of hydatidiform mole, subsequent pill use and the development of a trophoblastic tumour. The findings in relation to ovarian neoplasms is uncertain; as with ectopic pregnancy a long-term secular change in incidence cannot be discounted. Pill users are undoubtedly at a higher risk of liver tumours. Nonetheless, it *must* be remembered that the incidence of such tumours is exceedingly low; one estimate from the United States puts liver tumour incidence at 0·5 per 100 000 women in the whole population per annum (Vana *et al.*, 1977).

In conclusion, further rigorous epidemiological investigations are needed on a variety of sites in various populations to establish and, where relevant, quantify the additional risk or protective effect of pill use on the development of neoplasia of selected sites.

Pelvic inflammatory disease

As indicated earlier, the term pelvic inflammatory disease covers many forms of infection — and can include diverse conditions such as

Table VI
Risk factors: pill use and neoplasia

Neoplasm	Pill use	Risk factor compared with controls
Breast	Any use[a]	× 0·80
	2 + years[b]	× 0·25−0·80
Cervix[c]	3 + years	× 5 ??
Liver[d]	Continuously	
	5−7 years	× 5
	9 + years	× 25

Sources: [a] Vessey, 1979; [b] Population Reports, 1977; [c] Ory *et al.*, 1977; [d] Edmondson, Henderson and Benson, 1976.

gonorrhea, salpingitis and tubo-ovarian abscesses. Many such diseases *can* render the woman sterile; other forms of PID are milder, may be asymptomatic and end in spontaneous cure. PID is certainly more common in IUD users than in non-users, although estimates of the size of the risk vary substantially from 2 to 10 (Guillebaud, 1978; Population Reports, 1979). One American writer put the figure at 4·4 (Eschenbach *et al.*, 1977). In Sweden, Weström has shown that nulliparous users were *seven* times as likely to develop PID as nulliparous non-users. The corresponding figure for multiparous users was just under two (1·7) (Weström *et al.*, 1976).

The diagnosis and treatment of PID present substantial clinical problems. However, since there is widespread use of IUDs by single (generally never-pregnant) women, it is essential to consider the possible effect of PID on subsequent fertility. Weström followed up 415 women with laparoscopically proven PID. These women were studied for 14 years, and compared with a control group who had never developed PID. Twenty-one per cent of his PID cases were subsequently sterile compared with 3 per cent of the control group (tubal occlusion was not the reason for sterility in the control group). One in eight women had blocked tubes after one episode of infection, and three in four after 3 episodes (Weström, 1975). There are, therefore, considerable practical implications for clinicians when advising young women who plan to use this method of contraception. The matter of PID and ectopic pregnancy is discussed in the next section.

Ectopic pregnancy

Ectopic pregnancy, whatever its cause, remains a matter of major concern to the patient and her doctor. Unless swiftly and expertly treated it can result in death. Beral has documented the secular increase in ectopic pregnancy in England and Wales over the past 30 or so years (Beral, 1975). Sivin has reported a rise in the United States from 14 900 in 1965 to 40 700 in 1977; the associated incidence has more than doubled (Table VII) (Sivin, 1979). The reader should note that these figures are related to *women*, not to pregnancies. Undoubtedly, ectopic pregnancy occurring with the device *in situ*, ectopic pregnancy following abortion or failed sterilization and ectopic pregnancy whilst taking progestogen-only therapy have all contributed to the rising pattern. Nonetheless, it is impossible to discount an increased true incidence of ectopic conceptions. (For more detailed discussion see Beral, 1975 and Sivin, 1979.)

Users of intra-uterine devices are at higher risk of tubal implantation

Table VII
Ectopic pregnancies in the United States

Year	Number of ectopic pregnancies amongst women aged 15−44	Rate per 1000 women aged 15−44
1965	14 900	0·38
1968	18 700	0·46
1971	19 300	0·44
1974	26 800	0·58
1977	40 700	0·83

Source: Sivin, 1979.

than non-users. The factor is put variously at between 6 and 10 times as high (Seward *et al.*, 1972; Vessey *et al.*, 1974; Perlmutter, 1978). Two theories have been advanced. Lehfeldt and his colleagues have argued that the IUD is less successful at preventing ectopic pregnancy than it is at preventing its uterine counterpart. In 1970 they suggested that the IUD prevented 99·5 per cent of uterine pregnancies, 95 per cent of tubal ones, and had no effect on ovarian pregnancies (Lehfeldt, *et al.*, 1970). There is some support from Finland for this approach (Savolainen and Saksela, 1978). The alternative proposition — not mutually exclusive with the first — suggested that IUD-related inflammation interferes with the transport of the fertilized ovum (Tatum and Schmidt, 1977). A duration-of-use effect has also been identified in IUD users; the ratio of ectopic to uterine pregnancies increases with duration of use (Vessey *et al.*, 1974; Tatum *et al.*, 1976). These data are difficult to interpret since there is a definable age effect in relation to the incidence of ectopic pregnancies anyway (Savolainen and Saksela, 1978).

If the incidence of ectopic pregnancies in a non-contracepting population is taken to be about 1 in 250 pregnancies; then the corresponding incidence for IUD user failures is between about 1 in 25 and 1 in 60 pregnancies. Weström, in the study cited on PID and subsequent fertility, found that one in 24 pregnancies in his group were ectopic. Thus it is possible that following infection and after discontinuing with the device, the chance of an ectopic pregnancy is extremely high — somewhere near the maximum figure for the probability after a failure with the IUD *in situ*. The figures here should be treated with great caution, since no attempt can be made to match the characteristics of the groups covered in the various studies.

Recently Sivin (1979) has reported a significant increase of ectopic pregnancies between the second and third years of use of the Copper T device. If these findings are substantiated by other workers, two worrying questions must be faced. Firstly, it is only relatively recently that users have been advised to retain their devices for longer than two years. Sivin's finding could mean that the *number* of ectopic implantations will increase. And secondly, these and other data related to increased duration of use, suggest that it is timely to examine the issues of pregnancy, PID and subsequent fertility in those women who have had more than one device inserted consecutively.

Cardiovascular disease

The excess mortality from this cause is now a well accepted phenomenon. For this reason it is covered only briefly in this chapter. For information a summary table of the major risk factors has been included (Table VIII). The major sources of data on which this conclusion has been reached are the two prospective studies undertaken in the

Table VIII
Risk factors for mortality from diseases of the circulatory system; pill users and controls

		Risk factors (ratio of death-rates in user categories to controls)		
		Ever-user	Current user	Ex-user
All diseases of the circulatory system		4.7[b]	4.9[b]	4.3[b]
Non-rheumatic heart-disease and hypertension		4.0[c]	4.7[c]	3.0
Cerebrovascular disease		4.7[c]	4.4	5.3
Age	25−34	2.0		
All diseases of the circulatory system	35−44	4.5[c]		
Smoking[a]	No	4.7		
All diseases of the circulatory system	Yes	4.4[b]		
Duration of use (months)	1−59	3.4		
All diseases of the circulatory system	60 +	9.7		

[a] Actual death rates per 100 000 woman-years: non-smoker ever-user 13.8 (5); non-smoker control 3.0 (2); smoker ever-user 39.5 (19); smoker control 8.9 (3). (The number in brackets is the number of women in the sample.)

[b] $p < 0.01$.

[c] $p < 0.05$.

Source: Royal College of General Practitioners, 1977.

United Kingdom, one by the Royal College of General Practitioners and the other the Oxford Family Planning Association group. Death-rates from diseases of the circulatory system (covering a wide variety of vascular conditions) in the Royal College of General Practitioners' study were found to be higher by a factor of 5 in pill users as compared with non-user controls. An age-effect was demonstrated, as was a 'smoking' effect: these two factors are thought to act synergistically as opposed to additively. A duration-of-use effect was also evident — the risk factor rising to 10 amongst women who had used the pill continuously for five or more years (Table VIII) (Royal College of General Practitioners, 1977). These findings were supported by the Oxford Study (Vessey *et al.*, 1977).

Although we do not wish in any way to doubt the credence of the excess mortality experienced by pill users, it is important to remember the small numbers upon which these conclusions are based. In the first study cited there were 29 deaths — 16 among users, eight among ex-users and five in the controls; in the Oxford study there were nine deaths among users and none amongst the controls. Tietze recently reviewed these findings in the light of the American experience. He stated that a risk factor of between four and five was not consistent with the United States mortality statistics, and went on to add that "epidemiological studies based on small numbers may result in imprecise answers as to the *level* of risk" (Tietze, 1979). Both he and the authors of the two studies questioned the applicability of the risk level across societies.

There has also been some recent controversy regarding the use of vital statistics data to interpret trends in cardiovascular disease in relation to pill use and smoking (Beral, 1976; Belsey, *et al.*, 1979). Although these data — and the conclusions drawn from them — are in themselves interesting, we do not feel that they can be accepted as a basic approach to the study of subjects such as this.

ABORTION

The numbers of terminations of pregnancy performed under the 1967 Abortion Act rose steadily each year from 1968 onwards. A peak was reached in 1973, when just over 169 000 abortions were performed. Since 1973, however, the numbers have declined, and in 1976 the number of operations was nearly 128 000. Abortions performed on women who are not resident in England and Wales have also fallen substantially, from 56 000 in 1973 to under 28 000 in 1976. Forty per cent of operations are carried out in National Health Service (NHS) premises; and almost all of these are performed on residents of England

and Wales. When we examine the characteristics of residents who undergo termination of pregnancy we find that approximately half are single, 40 per cent are married and the remaining ten per cent belong to the 'other' marital status group (Table IX). Single women have generally never had a previous live birth and they are aged less than 25; married women are usually over 25 and have had at least two previous live births. The two categories — nulliparous single women aged under 25, and married women of over 25 with two or more previous births — account for nearly two-thirds of all abortions on resident women (Table IX).

Data on gestation of pregnancy at termination are shown in Table X. 80 per cent of operations are performed in the first twelve weeks of pregnancy. The proportion is slightly higher in the non-NHS sector — 84 per cent compared with the NHS figure of 77 per cent. The proportion of *very* early abortions — done at less than 9 weeks gestation — is significantly higher in the private sector — 33 per cent compared with 17 per cent in the NHS. Although the public sector undoubtedly performs more of the difficult and complex operations, these data suggest quite strongly that private organizations process their clients to abortion more swiftly than does the Health Service. Only one per cent of abortions are

Table IX
Legal abortions, England and Wales 1976, by age, marital status and number of previous liveborn children, residents only.

	Number of previous liveborn children			
Age	0	1	2 +	Total
Single women				
< 25	37 871	2 491	555	40 917
25 +	6 136	1 286	738	8 160
Total	44 007	3 777	1 293	49 077[a]
Married women				
< 25	1 822	1 876	2 885	6 583
25 +	2 256	3 938	26 502	32 696
Total	4 078	5 814	29 387	39 279[b]

[a] 1824 single women with age and/or number of previous liveborn children not stated have been excluded from the table.

[b] 1032 married women with age and/or number of previous liveborn children not stated have been excluded from the table.

An additional 10 700 women of other marital status have not been included.

Source: Office of Population Censuses and Surveys, 1979.

Table X
Legal abortions, England and Wales, 1976; by gestation and type of premises, residents only.

Gestation in weeks	Type of premises					
	NHS		Non-NHS		All	
< 9	8 475	(16·8)	16 761	(32·7)	25 236	(24·8)
9–12	30 685	(60·7)	26 184	(51·0)	56 869	(55·8)
13–16	7 509	(14·9)	5 542	(10·8)	13 051	(12·8)
17–19	1 068	(2·1)	1 153	(2·3)	2 221	(2·2)
20 +	450	(0·9)	525	(1·0)	975	(1·0)
Not stated	2 382	(4·7)	1 178	(2·3)	3 560	(3·5)
Total	50 569	(100·1)	51 343	(100·1)	101 912	(100·1)

Figures in parentheses are percentages.
Source: Office of Population Censuses and Surveys, 1979.

performed at, or after, 20 weeks of pregnancy, and both the numbers and percentages are the same for the two abortion-providing sectors — one per cent of the total and about 500 operations in each sector per annum.

The conventionally classified complications associated with termination of pregnancy are sepsis and haemorrhage. Other problems can include damage to pelvic organs, embolism, circulatory problems etc. The incidence of complications is shown in Table XI. Sepsis and haemorrhage are treated separately, and all other complications are grouped together in one category. The data have been presented separately for abortion alone and abortion with sterilization. This latter group accounted for 8900 operations, or 8·7 per cent of all procedures in 1976. Two groups of *types* of operation have been presented: vacuum aspiration, dilation and evacuation or some combination of the two; and all other methods (which includes, for example, prostaglandins, saline, etc.). The first group of methods is more often than not associated with first trimester abortions, and the second group with operations performed later in pregnancy. Complication rates increase from 8 per 1000 operations in the first twelve weeks of pregnancy to 36 per 1000 at thirteen weeks or later. First trimester abortions performed by vacuum aspiration and/or dilation and evacuation have a complication rate of under 6 per 1000 procedures, whilst later abortions performed by other methods have an associated figure of 81 per 1000 procedures.

Rates of complications increase substantially with the first category of

Table XI

Legal abortion, England and Wales, 1976; complication rates (gestation and method specific) per 1000 operations; abortion alone and abortion with sterilization, residents only.

(a) Abortion only

Gestation (in weeks)	Complication	Method		
		Vacuum aspiration, dilation and evacuation, alone or in combination	All other methods	Total
<13	Sepsis	0·9	2·4	0·9
	Haemorrhage	1·6	9·0	1·8
	Other	3·2	92·7	5·2
	Total	5·7	104·1	7·9
	(No. of complications)	(418)	(174)	(592)
	(No. of abortions)	(73 149)	(1 672)	(74 999)
13+	Sepsis	2·0	1·6	1·8
	Haemorrhage	4·2	4·7	4·4
	Other	7·1	74·7	30·2
	Total	13·3	81·0	36·4
	(No. of complications)	(129)	(411)	(540)
	(No. of abortions)	(9 716)	(5 075)	(14 853)
All gestations	Sepsis	1·0	1·8	1·1
	Haemorrhage	2·0	5·8	2·3
	Other	3·8	76·8	9·4
	Total	6·8	84·4	12·8
	(No. of complications)	(577)	(608)	(1 185)
	(No. of abortions)	(85 544)	(7 205)	(93 003)

(b) *Abortion with sterilization*

Gestation (in weeks)	Complication	Method		
		Vacuum aspiration, dilation and evacuation, alone or in combination	All other methods	Total
<13	Sepsis	2·1	7·6	2·8
	Haemorrhage	4·2	21·7	6·5
	Other	7·5	41·3	11·8
	Total	13·8	70·7	21·1
	(No. of complications)	(85)	(65)	(150)
	(No. of abortions)	(6 152)	(920)	(7 106)
13+	Sepsis	5·0	3·8	4·3
	Haemorrhage	6·6	15·3	11·5
	Other	11·6	28·1	20·8
	Total	23·2	47·2	36·6
	(No. of complications)	(14)	(37)	(51)
	(No. of abortions)	(604)	(784)	(1 394)
All gestations	Sepsis	2·4	5·5	3·0
	Haemorrhage	4·3	18·7	7·2
	Other	7·9	35·3	13·5
	Total	14·6	59·5	23·7
	(No. of complications)	(103)	(108)	(211)
	(No. of abortions)	(7 053)	(1 815)	(8 909)

Cases not stated have been included in the marginal totals, so that rows/columns do not necessarily add to their totals.
Source: Office of Population Censuses and Surveys, 1979.

operative procedures (vacuum aspiration, etc.) if a sterilization is performed in association with the termination of pregnancy — from 6 to 14 per 1000 with the first trimester operations, and from 13 to 23 with second trimester pregnancies. For 'other' methods, however, the reverse is true; complication rates decline from 104 to 71 (at less than 13 weeks of pregnancy) and from 81 to 60 (at 13 or more weeks).

More than 5000 abortions in NHS facilities and just under 11 000 operations in the non-NHS sector were performed on an outpatient basis, that is without an overnight stay, in 1976.

Mortality from legal abortion has continued to decline. Table XII demonstrates that the death-rate has fallen consistently since 1969. The rate is now less than 1 per 100 000 operations. Death-rates are in fact higher in the NHS premises (Office of Population Censuses and Surveys, 1979). This presumably reflects in part the lower proportion of early, and therefore relatively safer, abortions performed in them in comparison with the private sector of care. However, it should be noted that three of the abortion deaths in NHS premises between 1973 and 1975 were transfers from private nursing homes after post-operative complications had developed (Department of Health and Social Security, 1979). Deaths from illegal and spontaneous abortions are discussed in the next section.

For some 8000 women the termination of pregnancy performed in 1976 was the second such operation which they had undergone under the provisions of the Abortion Act. A little under half the women were

Table XII
Deaths from legal abortion, numbers and rates, by types of premises in which they occurred: England and Wales, 1969–76.

Year	Type of premises			Rate per 100 000 legal abortions[a]
	NHS	Non-NHS	Total	
1969	14	3	17	31·0
1970	14	–	14	16·2
1971	10	4	14	11·0
1972	13	2	15	9·4
1973	4	2	6	3·6
1974	5	2	7	4·3
1975	2	1	3	2·1
1976	1	–	1	0·8

[a] Ratio of all deaths to total legal abortions performed.
Source: Office of Population Censuses and Surveys, 1979.

single. One disturbing feature of the figures is that 64 girls aged under 16 in 1976 were presenting for termination of an unwanted pregnancy for the second time. However, the increasing number of repeat abortions can be expected and reflects the increasing number of women in the population who have had a first abortion, and who are, therefore, at risk of a second abortion. Tietze has argued that an increase may occur even when contraceptive practice improves (Tietze, 1978; Tietze and Jain, 1978).

The psychological sequelae of abortion have been reported in detail, and studies have originated in both the pro- and anti-abortion segments of the community. Effects range from the negligible to (occasional) admission to a mental hospital during a psychotic episode (Illsley and Hall, 1976; Deven, 1976; Brewer, 1977). There are also a few studies on the children born to women after abortion has been refused. The most recently published of these appeared last year and is based on Czechoslovakian data (Matejcek et al., 1978). The authors conclude that "although differences between wanted and control children were not dramatic, they were consistent and multiple and tend to support the major hypothesis that the development of children born of unwanted pregnancies would be more problem prone".

STERILIZATION

Sterilization — male and female — is being increasingly used, in all parts of the world, as the means for controlling fertility when desired family size has been reached. In the United States there are about 600 000 male and 600 000 female operations each year (Hulka, 1978). In fact, results from the 1975 National Fertility Survey show that one or other partner in *half* the couples who were white, had been continuously married for 10 or more years and who were practising contraception had undergone a sterilization procedure (Westoff and Jones, 1977). Data are not so easy to come by for the United Kingdom. Bone recently estimated that six per cent of wives and six per cent of husbands in couples where the wife was ever-married and aged under 45 had been sterilized (Bone, 1978a). These figures relate to England and Wales. A corresponding annual figure of 33 000 operations comes from another source, but is now well out of date since it relates to 1971 (Department of Health and Social Security, 1974). More information on female sterilization is available for Scotland, where there were about 13 500 operations in 1976 (Teper and Clarke, 1979; Clarke, 1979). It has also been established that certain areas of Scotland have had a relatively extensive resort to sterilization over a long period of time (Teper, 1978). General figures for vasectomy in the United Kingdom are not immediately available.

There are a number of standard techniques used in operations to sterilize a woman. Until ten years ago *laparotomy* was the usual approach. This involves major abdominal surgery, general anaesthesia, and a hospital stay usually of several days. Although generally it is not the operation of choice in developed societies, it remains important because of its relevance in other societies. *Laparoscopy* has been increasingly refined as a technique, and is now extensively used in Britain, America and in many other countries throughout the world (including some Third World countries). Laparoscopic sterilization can be performed in a few minutes, and general anaesthesia and a hospital stay are not always necessary. The technique, however, is extremely sophisticated in terms of its demands on surgical skills and equipment maintenance. It still remains a procedure with significant morbidity from complications. An alternative endoscopic technique — *culdoscopy* — is used in some areas. This uses a vaginal as opposed to an abdominal approach. The technique of *minilaparotomy* has been pioneered by some surgeons, who feel that laparoscopy is an over-complex technique: it has gained particular acceptance in areas where it is impossible to maintain adequately the sophisticated and expensive equipment needed for laparoscopic sterilization (Schima *et al.*, 1974; Schima and Lubell, 1976; Connell, 1978).

As might be expected, it is possible to derive a wide range of failure rates which vary by technique, population characteristics, operator and various other parameters. Some results from an international follow-up of 8500 women are shown in Table XIII. Six-month life table pregnancy rates were highest in women who underwent sterilization after abortion and lowest following interval sterilization. Clip sterilization had a higher failure rate than other techniques of tubal occlusion. It is disturbing to note that half the failures after electro-coagulation were ectopic pregnancies (McCann and Kessel, 1978). Failure rates with any method of tubal occlusion or destruction can be expected to improve over time as more general experience is gained and as individual surgeons develop their own expertise.

Operative complications reported have ranged between 0·1 and about 13 per 1000 procedures; correspondingly morbidity figures of between 0·5 and 3·0 per cent have been presented (Cummins, 1976). When complications occur during laparoscopy they can be dramatic — and fatal. Whichever technique is selected for sterilization, death can occur; the confidential enquiry on maternal deaths discussed in the next section notes that 12 deaths occurred with all types of

Table XIII
Six-month and twelve-month life table pregnancy rates (per 100 women) following laparoscopic sterilization, by timing of operation and method of tubal occlusion/destruction

Timing of operation (number of cases in parentheses)	Cases		Method of tubal destruction/ occlusion	Rate per 100 women[a]	
	6-months	12-months		6-month	12-month
Interval	4 326	2 080	Electro-coagulation	0·2 (0·1)	0·4 (0·1)
	1 257	872	Clip	0·9 (0·6)	2·2 (0·7)
	1 519	676	Ring	0·2 (0·1)	0·6 (0·3)
Post-abortion	243	—	Electro-coagulation	0·7 (0·6)	—
	171	—	Clip	2·6 (1·3)	—
	360	—	Ring	0·0 (0·0)	—
Post-partum	252	246	Electro-coagulation	0·4 (0·5)	0·4 (0·5)

[a] Standard errors are in parentheses
Source: McCann and Kessel, 1978

sterilization in England and Wales in the three-year period 1973−75.

The existence of the phenomenon of post-sterilization menorrhagia has yet to be scientifically established. Long-term use of oral contraception may mean that a woman becomes unfamiliar with the pattern of her own 'normal' cycle.

The majority of women appear to be satisfied with the operation (Schima and Lubell, 1976), although there is some evidence that some surgeons — and their patients — make unwise decisions (Winston, 1977).

In the past two or three years there has been a growing interest in the possibility of reversal. Some gynaecologists no longer regard the operation as 'permanent' and are prepared to attempt reversal. Some advocate the use of those techniques most likely to offer reversibility for use with those patients perceived to be at high risk of requesting reanastamosis (Hulka, 1978). Subsequent pregnancy cannot, of course, be guaranteed.

Vasectomy — male sterilization — is a straightforward and safe procedure. It is particularly suitable for those whose families are complete. It has been known to be successfully performed in a variety of venues, ranging from general practitioners' surgeries to railway stations. The main contra-indications to the operation are local infections and systemic blood disorders. The side-effects which occur most frequently are swelling, pain and discoloration of the skin. These events are harmless and disappear within a few days or weeks at most (Morgan, 1972; Blandy, 1973). More serious problems encountered include haematoma (Davis, 1972), infection (infrequent), sperm granuloma and epididymitis. All these are relatively infrequent and respond well to treatment where necessary. No systemic effects have yet been identified in vasectomized men. Failure rates appear to be at or less than 1 per 100 procedures (Davis and Shulman, 1974). On occasions spontaneous recanalization occurs, but this happens rarely; one worker has put its occurrence at less than a quarter of one per cent of cases (Leader et al., 1974). Failure is a function of the technique used, and sometimes a structure other than the vas is ligated. A few men suffer psychological side-effects after the operation, but these are often found to be men who had sexual disturbances prior to vasectomy (Schima et al., 1974; Schima and Lubell, 1976).

As with female sterilization, the issue of reversibility has become a topic for discussion. Such operations are now performed with some degree of success. Frozen semen storage prior to vasectomy is also now a reality. A review of the material on vasovasostomy up to and including 1976 is available in Population Reports, 1976 and a general discussion is available in Hulka (1978) (see also Schima et al., 1974; Schima and Lubell, 1976).

CHILDBIRTH

Maternal mortality — deaths during pregnancy, childbirth and in the puerperium — are monitored in England, Wales and Scotland by the continuing process of the *confidential enquiry* into such deaths. Reports on the topic are published regularly for England and Wales, and separately for Scotland. A distinction is drawn between *true* maternal deaths and those which are termed *associated*. Full details of definitions, statistical aspects, etc are available in publications by the Department of Health and Social Security (1979), and the Scottish Home and Health Department (1978). Only *true* maternal deaths are discussed here.

The most recent report for England and Wales covers the period 1973–75. During the three years 235 true maternal deaths were reported. The Office of Population Censuses and Surveys identified a further 19 true maternal deaths, five of which related to abortion, which were not included in the confidential enquiry. The 235 deaths correspond to a death-rate of 12·2 per 100 000 *maternities*, or 10·7 if deaths from all types of abortion are excluded. These compare with rates of

15·5 and 11·9 respectively per 100 000 maternities in the preceding period 1970–72. The general downward trend in maternal mortality, therefore, continued. Data made available last year show a slight increase in maternal mortality for 1976 and 1977 (Department of Health and Social Security, 1978).

The main causes of maternal deaths are shown in Table XIV. As a single group of causes, hypertensive diseases account for the largest number (39) followed by pulmonary embolism (35); and then haemorrhage, ectopic pregnancy and sepsis (21 each). Abortion (of all forms) accounted for 29 deaths in the three-year period. There has been a decline in each cause category in comparison with the previous period. Particular progress has been made in relation to abortion — where the death-*rate* was more than halved between 1970–72 and 1973–75, pulmonary embolism — with a 30 per cent fall in the death-rate, and ectopic pregnancy — with a decline of 26 per cent. Although there was a small numerical fall in the numbers of deaths in both categories, little progress has been made in reducing the death-*rates* from haemorrhage and hypertensive diseases.

Of the 29 abortion deaths ten were classified as resulting from illegal abortion (either criminal or self-induced), five were as a result of

Table XIV
Causes of true maternal deaths (i.e. directly related to pregnancy or childbirth); England and Wales, 1973–75.

Cause	Number of deaths
Pulmonary embolism	35
Haemorrhage	21
Hypertensive diseases of pregnancy	39
Sepsis[a]	21
Amniotic fluid embolism	14
Ruptured uterus	11
Ectopic pregnancy	21
Other	44
Total	206[b]
Abortion	29
Total	235[b]

[a] Excludes abortion with sepsis and ectopic pregnancy with sepsis.
[b] A further 14 unreported maternal and 5 abortion deaths were identified by the Office of Population Censuses and Surveys.
Source: Department of Health and Social Security, 1979.

spontaneous abortion, and the remaining 14 were from legal abortions. This latter figure of 14 deaths for 1973 – 75 differs by 2 from the figures in Table XII. This reflects the distinction made in the confidential enquiries between true and associated deaths (Department of Health and Social Security, 1979).

During the process of examining individual case histories responsibility, when appropriate, is allocated to the medical practitioner or to the patient, and the death classified as 'avoidable' or not. An avoidable death is one in which alternative management might have resulted in a better outcome. The involvement of doctors and patients in some of the deaths is shown in Table XV. Nearly three-quarters of the deaths from hypertensive diseases and haemorrhage might have had a better outcome had the clinicians involved acted differently; up to 30 per cent of these cases also included some element of patient non-compliance. The report emphasizes the necessity for appropriate clinical management; both in relation to swift admission to hospital when necessary, and to the need for *experienced* obstetric staff to be on hand. This latter point is stressed more than once in the report. The characteristics of those women who are particularly at risk of specific complications are reiterated (see the last column of Table XV).

Discussion

It is perhaps not surprising that a review of the risks and hazards associated with fertility control results in a rather dispiriting picture. After all, if one sets out to find medical problems in this area one is likely to find them. Nevertheless, it is important to retain a realistic perspective against which to examine the issues. And it is particularly important to remember that all forms of medication (and indeed all forms of surgery) carry with them the risk of an adverse effect. Even the humble aspirin — for example — has been known to produce asthmatic attacks in susceptible individuals (Laurence, 1966).

Despite the somewhat gloomy arguments of the preceding pages, there are reasonable contraceptive options open to many women. Oral contraception remains appropriate for those aged under 35 — some would say 30 — especially if they are non-smokers and do not have weight problems. The IUD certainly has a place in the contraceptive armamentarium, although the problems of PID may make it more suitable as a technique for married women who wish to space their pregnancies than for unmarried nulliparous women who may have several

Table XV

Selected items of information on maternal deaths: England and Wales, 1973–75.

Cause	Approximate percentage of deaths classified as 'avoidable'[a]	Approximate percentage of 'avoidable' cases in which patient implicated	Clinical implications	Risk groups
Hypertensive diseases	74	17	Vigilance in early detection and treatment	35+ 'prims, para 4+, non-Caucasian
Haemorrhage	71	28	Urgent hospital admission, use of obstetric flying squad, use of experienced surgeons	30+, para 3 or 4+
Pulmonary embolism	30	27	—	30+, para 4+, Caesarean section.

[a] i.e. different action by doctor and/or patient might have produced better outcome.

Source: Department of Health and Social Security, 1979.

sexual partners. For long-term limitation sterilization procedures for either partner may be acceptable, and carry with them relatively low rates of morbidity and mortality.

Tietze and others (1976) have shown that the use of barrier methods of contraception combined with early abortion is, in terms of mortality, the safest contraceptive regimen for women — irrespective of the age at which they initiate contraceptive practice. To put this approach forward for use in Britain would seem to be an act of social and political folly. At a personal level several early abortions during the reproductive life-span would not be acceptable to many women. In addition, the demand for abortion would be substantial, and it is probably unreasonable to expect gynaecologists to undertake that kind of alteration in their work-load.

In his calculations Tietze estimated the mortality risks from any single contraceptive method used over the whole child-bearing period from the initiation of contraception. This represents a simplification of individual experience. Bone (1978b) and others have shown that women and couples frequently have experience of more than one method. There is urgent need for computations of risk which reflect the most frequently adopted patterns of contraception used by an individual or couple over a period of time, and which examine not only contraceptive failure and mortality but also patterns of morbidity.

Research for new methods of contraception remains a priority. At the same time it is important that available methods which are not widely used in this country be assessed for use here, or for use on a broader scale than obtains at present. The progestogen-only pill could very well be a good contraceptive option for some women, and it would be sensible to undertake controlled trials in this country. The limited literature on Depo-Provera used in the United Kingdom makes disappointing reading; this is partly because it is often used for groups of the population who are perceived as being the least able to use other forms of contraception successfully, and who are the least likely to create and use opportunities for communicating problems which occur during use of the substance (Wilson, 1976; Savage, 1978).

Although it seems an obvious point to make, it is imperative to stress the need for adequate supervision of women using contraceptive methods which carry risks of morbidity. For example, clinicians must be aware of the risks of liver tumours and ectopic pregnancies. This has serious implications for the continuing education of general practitioners and family planning doctors. There may well be risks associated with currently available methods which are as yet undiscovered. A recent review on oral contraception, for example, listed 116 biochemical effects (Briggs and Briggs, 1977, 1978). It is also important that clinicians develop the skills of communicating factual information to their clients. The tools of health education have a real role to play here (Department of Health and Social Security, 1977).

Having reviewed the literature in this field, perhaps the most important implications appear to relate to service provision, especially in terms of abortion, sterilization and obstetric services. Despite the decline in the numbers of abortions performed each year, the level of the resort to legally induced termination of pregnancy continues to be substantial. Greater use of the more efficient means of birth control and more efficient use of other techniques do not mean, of necessity, less abortion. It is therefore of vital importance that whenever abortions are performed they are performed as early in gestation as possible, and facilities must be made available to this end. The proportion of out-patient abortions in this country is still quite low. The issues involved in day-care units are complex (Pregnancy Advisory Service, 1974) but there is scope for reducing the costs of the procedure to the Health Service and for minimizing stress for individuals who seek this particular outcome of pregnancy.

Some of the same factors apply to sterilization. In many parts of the world these operations are successfully completed under local anaesthesia and on an ambulatory basis. Although this will not be appropriate in every case the various merits and demerits of the individual approaches — both in relation to specific technique and to the use of anaesthesia — need a sound evaluation in order to make the best use of available resources. The development of methods with a greater likelihood of reversibility makes sterilization a less final option. None the less, with the present state of technology, it would be unfortunate if reversibility became an expectation of couples who are seeking to undergo the procedure.

In terms of obstetric services, the recent reports on maternal mortality are reasonably encouraging. However, in comparison with other countries there is no room for complacency. This is especially true in relation to the Scandinavian countries. (See Table XVI.) The data in Table XVI are expressed as rates per 100 000 live births, not per 100 000 *maternities* and are not exactly comparable with those discussed above. If the rate of about 5 maternal deaths per 100 000 births obtaining in Denmark, Norway and Sweden had applied here, then only 95 women would have died in England and Wales in the period 1973−75 compared to the actual toll of 235 lives. It is frequently argued that very different standards of living and of health care exist in Scandinavia. When we examine the data for England and Wales by region we find

Table XVI
Number of live births, maternal deaths and abortion deaths, and maternal death-rates
(including deaths from abortion); selected countries 1972–75.

Country	Births	Numbers of deaths		Average maternal death-rate (including abortion) per 100 000 live births[b]
		Maternal	Abortion	
Denmark[a]	218 727	10	1	4·6 (4·1)
Sweden	435 231	21	–	4·8
Norway[a]	185 071	10	–	5·4
Finland[a]	177 788	16	4	9·0 (6·7)
Israel[a]	267 255	26	3	9·7 (8·6)
Netherlands	772 980	88	4	11·4 (10·9)
Canada[a]	1 034 337	125	5	12·1 (11·6)
England & Wales[c]	1 939 010	220	34	13·1 (11·3)
Switzerland	341 831	56	10	16·4 (13·5)
Scotland	290 978	51	7	17·5 (15·1)
France[a]	2 536 424	605	98	23·9 (20·0)
Ireland[a]	204 419	51	4	25·0 (23·0)

[a] 1972–74 data
[b] Rates excluding abortion are in brackets.
[c] 1973–75 data — includes deaths identified by OPCS but not included in the Confidential Enquiries.
Source: Scottish Home and Health Department, 1978, Department of Health and Social Security, 1979.

that there are areas which have achieved extremely low maternal death-rates. Oxford for example has a rate of 4·4; and although the region may be said to be relatively 'privileged', the same cannot be said of the Trent region. Trent is industrialized, has a high rate of illegitimacy and poor health spending — and a maternal mortality rate of about half the national average at 6·0. At the other end of the scale Wessex has a rate of 16·8 and North East Thames of 18·6. These regional rates are true maternal mortality rates *excluding* abortion. We should also note that although France appears to have made great strides with her level of perinatal mortality, the same cannot be said of her maternal mortality (Table XVI). But the most important issue arising from the present pattern of maternal mortality is that the limitations of the services which contribute to the 'avoidability' factor of maternal deaths must inevitably contribute in a causal way to unnecessary morbidity amongst women being delivered of their infants. Since women are actively discouraged from giving birth in non-hospital environments, inadequate obstetric services and lack of skilled and experienced medical staff represent a situation which is unacceptable at both the practical and political level.

Finally, mention should be made of the situation in Third World countries. Although at first sight this may appear to be a digression from the main contents of this paper, there are two important reasons for the inclusion of at least a brief coverage here. First, there has been little research on the applicability of risk factors to societies which differ radically in structure from the Western model. In the developing world patterns of diet, exposure to disease, smoking habits and life-style all differ significantly from those in Europe. The incidence of circulatory disease is low; heart attacks and venous thromboembolic disease are rare. Risk factors derived from the British studies on circulatory disease and oral contraception apparently cannot be applied to the American population; it would be extremely surprising if they were generally appropriate in Asia, India and Africa.

The second point is that the equation between family planning and health is quite different in Third World countries. Bangladesh, for example, has a maternal mortality rate of about 200 per 100 000 women. The level of pill associated deaths is likely to be about 5 to 10 per cent of this rate. The use of contraception in these societies undoubtedly reduces mortality and is vital to public health programmes. It is however, imperative that the methods of contraception which are made available have minimal health risks and that appropriate medical services exist to deal with complications which arise from their use. Excessive blood loss resulting in anaemia may cause additional debility in a poor and undernourished population — correspondingly oral contraception, by reducing menstrual flow, may in fact improve the health status of the population. Lactation is vital to child health in much of the Third World, and the use of contraceptive methods which reduce milk supply are obviously to be questioned. Populations in rural areas may be several days, rather than hours, away from hospital facilities. The treatment of uterine perforation of an IUD will thus occur later rather than sooner; and more often than not ectopic pregnancy will be fatal. Research on the levels and applicability of risk factors in developing societies is urgently needed, and the development and implementation of appropriate health strategies is also essential (World Health Organisation, 1978).

In Britain most sexually active individuals are going to use contraception at some time during their reproductive life-span. They need information, guidance and support to select and use successfully the right method for themselves; the relevant methods may well change as couples build, space and then complete their families. The guardians of that information, guidance and support are the members of the medical profession. For the two sides of the interface to interact successfully is one, if not perhaps the greatest, challenge which preventive medicine faces in Britain — and indeed throughout the world — in coming decades.

References

Alvior, G.T. (1973). Pregnancy outcome with removal of intrauterine device. *Obstetrics and Gynecology*, 41, 894–896.

Belsey, M.A., Russell, Y. and Kinnear, K. (1979). Cardiovascular disease and oral contraceptives: a reappraisal of vital statistics data. *International Family Planning Perspectives*, 5, 2–7.

Beral, V. (1975). An epidemiological study of recent trends in ectopic pregnancy. *British Journal of Obstetrics and Gynaecology*, 82, 775–782.

Beral, V. (1976). Cardiovascular-disease mortality trends and oral-contraceptive use in young women. *Lancet*, ii, 1047–1052.

Blandy, J.P. (1973). Vasectomy as a method of family limitation. *Midwife, Health Visitor and Community Nurse* 8, 161–165.

Bone, M. (1978a). Recent trends in sterilization. *Population Trends*, 13, 13–16. Office of Population Censuses and Surveys. London; HMSO.

Bone, M. (1978b). *The Family Planning Services: Changes and Effects*. London: HMSO.

Boston Collaborative Drug Surveillance Program (1973). Oral contraceptives and venous thromboembolic disease, surgically confirmed gallbladder disease, and breast tumours. *Lancet*, i, 1399–1409.

Boyce, J.G., Lu, T., Nelson, J.H. Jr. and Fruchter, R.G. (1977). Oral contraception and cervical carcinoma. *American Journal of Obstetrics and Gynecology*, 128, 761–766.

Brewer, C. (1977). Incidence of post-abortion psychosis: a prospective study. *British Medical Journal*, i, 476–477.

Briggs, M. and Briggs, M. (1977). *Oral Contraceptives*. Montreal: Eden Press.

Briggs, M. and Briggs, M. (1978). *Oral Contraceptives*, Vol. 2. Edinburgh: Churchill Livingstone.

British Medical Journal (1976). Editorial: Oral contraceptives and neoplasia. i, 545–546.

British Medical Journal (1977). Editorial: Liver tumours and the pill. ii, 345–346.

Cates, W. Jr., Ory, H.W., Rochat, R.W. and Tyler, C.W. Jr. (1976). The intrauterine device and deaths from spontaneous abortion. *New England Journal of Medicine*, 295, 1155–1159.

Clarke, J. (1979). Personal communication.

Cohen, C.J. and Deppe, G. (1977). Endometrial carcinoma and oral contraceptive agents. *Obstetrics and Gynecology*, 49, 390–392.

Connell, E. (1978). Female sterilization: the state of the art and future directions. *Contemporary Obstetrics and Gynecology*, 11. 111–115.

Cummins, G.T.M. (1976). An overview of female sterilization. In *New Advances in Sterilization*, edited by M.E. Schima and I. Lubell. New York: Association of Voluntary Sterilization.

Davis, J.E. (1972). Vasectomy. *American Journal of Nursing*, **72**, 509.

Davis, J.E. and Shulman, S. (1974). Male sterilization — clinical aspects. In *Advances in Voluntary Sterilization*, edited by M.E. Schima, I. Lubell, J.E. Davis and E. Connell. Amsterdam: Excerpta Medica; New York: Elsevier.

Department of Health and Social Security (1974). *On the State of the Public Health 1973*. London: HMSO.

Department of Health and Social Security (1977). *Prevention and Health, Reducing the Risk: Safer Pregnancy and Childbirth*. London: HMSO.

Department of Health and Social Security (1978). *On the State of the Public Health for the Year 1977*. London: HMSO.

Department of Health and Social Security (1979). *Report on Confidential Enquiries into Maternal Deaths in England and Wales 1973—1975*. Report on Health and Social Subjects 14. London: HMSO.

Deven, F. (1976). Review of psychosocial consequences of abortion. *Tijdschrift voor Sociale Wetenschappen*, **3**, 241—264.

Donnelly, P.K., Baker, K.W., Carney, J.A. and O'Fallon, W.M. (1975). Benign breast lesions and subsequent breast carcinoma in Rochester, Minnesota. *Mayo Clinic Proceedings*, **50**.

Edmondson, H.A., Henderson, B. and Benson, B. (1976). Liver-cell adenomas associated with use of oral contraceptives. *New England Journal of Medicine*, **294**, 470—472.

Emens, J.M., Gustafson, R.C. and Jordan, J.A. (1978). Early postpartum insertion of an intrauterine device. *Fertility and Contraception*, **2**, 38—41.

Eschenbach, D.A., Harnisch, J.P. and Holmes, K.K. (1977). Pathogenesis of acute pelvic inflammatory disease: role of contraception and other risk factors. *American Journal of Obstetrics and Gynecology*, **128**, 838—850.

Fasal, E. and Paffenbarger, R.S. (1975). Oral contraceptives related to cancer and benign lesions of the breast. *Journal of the National Cancer Institute*, **55**, 767—773.

Fisch, I.R. and Frank, J. (1977). Oral contraceptives and blood pressure. *Journal of the American Medical Association* **237**, 2499—2503.

Fotherby, K. (1977). Low doses of progestagens as fertility regulating agents. In *Regulation of Human Fertility*, edited by E. Diczfalusy. Copenhagen: Scriptor.

Guillebaud, J. (1978). Pelvic inflammatory disease and IUCDs. *British Journal of Family Planning*, **4**, 25.

Guillebaud, J., Bonnar, J., Morehead, J. and Matthews, A. (1976). Menstrual blood-loss with intrauterine devices. *Lancet*, **i**, 387—390.

Hulka, J.F. (1978). Current status of the reversibility of sterilization. *Research in Reproduction*, **10** (5), 1—2.

Hunton, M. (1976). A retrospective survey of over 1 000 patients on oral contraceptives in a group practice. *Journal of the Royal College of General Practitioners*, **26**, 538—546.

Illsley, R. and Hall, M.H. (1976). Psychosocial aspects of abortion. *Bulletin*, World Health Organisation, **53**, 83—106.

Ingemanson, C.A., Jägerhorn, M., Zizala, J., Nilsson, B. and Zador, G. (1976). Preliminary results from a Swedish multicentre trial of a new low dose combined oral contraceptive. *Acta Obstetrica et Gynecologica Scandinavica Supplement 54*.

Jain, A.K. and Moots, B. (1977). Fecundability following the discontinuation of IUD use among Taiwanese women. *Journal of Biosocial Science*, **9**, 137—151

Jain, A.K. and Sivin, I. (1977). Life-table analysis of IUDs: problems and recommendations. *Studies in Family Planning*, **8**, 25—47.

Kaulhausen, H. and Klingsiek, L. (1976). Clinical aspects of hypertension under contraceptive steroids. *Fortschrifte der Medizin*, **94**.

Keifer, W.S.Jr. and Scott, J.C. (1977). Liver neoplasma and the oral contraceptive. *American Journal of Obstetrics and Gynecology*, **128**, 448–454.

Laurence, D.R. (1966). *Clinical Pharmacology*. London: Churchill.

Leader, A.J., Axelrad, S.D., Frankowski, R. and Mumford, S.D. (1974). Complications of 2,711 vasectomies. *Journal of Urology*, **111**, 365–369.

Lehfeldt, H., Tietze, C. and Gorstein, F. (1970). Ovarian pregnancy and the intrauterine device. *American Journal of Obstetrics and Gynecology*, **108**, 1005–1009.

Lippes, J. (1978). Management of the lost IUD: a conservative approach. In *Risks, Benefits, and Controversies in Fertility Control*, edited by J.J. Sciarra, G.I. Zatuchni and J.J. Speidel. Hagerstown, Maryland: Harper & Row.

Livolsi, V.A., Stadel, B.V., Kelsey, J.L., Holford, T.R. and White, C. (1978). Fibrocystic breast disease in oral contraceptive users: a histopathological evaluation of epithelial atypia. *New England Journal of Medicine*, **299**, 381.

Luukkainen, T., Nielsen, N.-C., Nygren, K.-G., Pyörälä, T. and Allonen, H. (1979). Combined and national experience of post menstrual IUD insertions of Nova-T and Copper-T in a randomized study. *Contraception*, **19**, 11–20.

McCann, M.F. and Kessel, E. (1978). International experience with laparoscopic sterilization: a follow-up of 8500 women. *Advances in Planned Parenthood*, **12**, 199–211.

McEwan, J. (1977). Choosing which pill. *British Journal of Hospital Medicine*, **17**, 369–371.

MacLeod, J. and Tietze, C. (1964). Control of reproductive capacity. *Annual Review of Medicine*, **15**, 299–314.

Matejcek, Z., Dytrych, Z. and Schuller, V. (1978). Children from unwanted pregnancies. *Acta Psychiatrica Scandinavica*, **57**, Fasc. 1.

Monson, R.R., Yen, S., MacMahon, B. and Warren, S. (1976). Chronic mastitis and carcinoma of the breast. *Lancet*, **ii**, 224–226.

Morehead, J.E., Matthews, A., Guillebaud, J. and Bonnar, J. (1975). Menstrual blood loss in users of an IUD. In *Analysis of Intrauterine Contraception*, edited by F. Hefnawi and S.J. Segal. Amsterdam: North Holland; New York: American Elsevier.

Morgan, R.E. (1972). Vasectomy. *Pennsylvania Medicine*, **75**, 38–40.

Nilsson, C.G. (1977). Comparative quantitation of menstrual blood loss with a d-norgestrel-releasing IUD and a Nova-T-copper device. *Contraception*, **15**, 379–387.

Nissen, E.D., Kent, D.R. and Nissen, S.E. (1977). Etiologic factors in pathogenesis of liver tumours associated with oral contraception. *American Journal of Obstetrics and Gynecology*, **127**, 61–66.

Office of Population Censuses and Surveys (1979). *Abortion Statistics, 1976*. London: HMSO.

Ory, H. (1974). Functional ovarian cysts and oral contraceptives: negative association confirmed surgically: a cooperative study. *Journal of the American Medical Association*, **228**, 68.

Ory, H., Cole, P., MacMahon, B. and Hoover, R. (1976). Oral contraceptives and reduced risk of benign breast diseases. *New England Journal of Medicine*, **294**, 419.

Ory, H., Conger, S.B., Naib, Z., Tyler, C.W. and Hatcher, R.A. (1977). In *Pharmacology of Steroid and Contraceptive Drugs*, edited by S. Garattini and H.W. Berendes, H.W. New York: Raven Press.

Perlmutter, J.F. (1978). Pregnancy and the IUD. *Journal of Reproductive Medicine*, **20**,

133–138.

Population Reports (1976). *Sterilization*, Series D. No. 3. Washington, DC: George Washington University.

Population Reports (1977). *Oral Contraceptives*, Series A, No. 4. Washington, DC: George Washington University.

Population Reports (1979). *Intrauterine Devices*, Series B, No. 3. Washington DC: George Washington University.

Potter, R.G. (1966). Application of life table techniques to measurement of contraceptive effectiveness. *Demography*, 3, 297–304.

Pregnancy Advisory Service (1974). *Out-Patient Abortion*. London: Pregnancy Advisory Service.

Presser, H. (1971). The timing of the first birth, female roles and black fertility. *Milbank Memorial Fund Quarterly*, 49, 329–360.

Royal College of General Practitioners (1974). *Oral Contraceptives and Health*. London: Pitman.

Royal College of General Practitioners (1976). Oral contraception study: the outcome of pregnancy in former oral contraceptive users. *British Journal of Obstetrics and Gynaecology*, 83, 608–616.

Royal College of General Practitioners (1977). Oral contraceptive study: mortality among oral-contraceptive users. *Lancet*, ii, 727–731.

Ryder, N.B. (1973). Contraceptive failure in the United States. *Family Planning Perspectives*, 5, 133–142.

Savage, W. (1978). The use of Depo-Provera in East London. *Fertility and Contraception* 2, 41–47.

Savolainen, E. and Saksela, E. (1978). Ectopic pregnancy: relationship to the preceding contraception. *Annales Chirugiae et Gynaecologiae*, 67, 198–202.

Schima, M.E. and Lubell, I. (Editors) (1976). *New Advances in Sterilization*. New York: Association of Voluntary Sterilization.

Schima, M.E., Lubell, I., Davis, J.E. and Connell, E. (Editors) (1974). *Advances in Voluntary Sterilization*. Amsterdam: Excerpta Medica; New York: Elsevier.

Scottish Home and Health Department (1978). *A Report on an Enquiry Into Maternal Deaths in Scotland 1972–1975*. Edinburgh: HMSO.

Segal, S.J. and Tietze, C. (1971). Contraceptive technology: current and prospective methods. *Reports on Population/Family Planning*, 1, 1–20.

Seward, P.N., Israel, R. and Ballard, C.A. (1972). Ectopic pregnancy and intrauterine contraception: a definite relationship. *Obstetrics and Gynecology*, 40, 214–217.

Shine, R.M. and Thompson, J.F. (1974). The in situ IUD and pregnancy. *American Journal of Obstetrics and Gynecology*, 119, 124–130.

Sivin, I. (1979). Copper T IUD use and ectopic pregnancy rates in the United States. *Contraception*, 19, 151–173.

Snowden, R., Williams, M. and Hawkins, D. (1977). *The IUD: A Practical Guide*. London: Croom Helm.

Soutoul, J.-H., Renaud, M., Jallatte, C.S. and Bertrand, J. (1976). Oral contraception by means of progestagen-only micropills taken continuously in the light of four recent trials. *Revue Francaise de Gynecologie et L'Obstetrique*, 71, 761–773.

Stone, M., Dent, J., Kardana, A. and Bagshawe, K.D. (1976). Relationship of oral contraception to development of trophoblastic tumour after evacuation of hydatidiform mole. *British Journal of Obstetrics and Gynaecology*, 83, 913–916.

Stopes, M.C. (1925). *The First Five Thousand*. London: John Bale, Sons & Danielsson.

Tatum, H.J. (1977). Clinical aspects of intrauterine contraception: circumspection

1976. *Fertility and Sterility*, **28**, 3−28.

Tatum, H.J. and Schmidt, F.H. (1977). Contraceptive and sterilization practices and extrauterine pregnancy: a realistic perspective. *Fertility and Sterility*, **28**, 407−421.

Tatum, H.J., Schmidt, F.H. and Jain, A.K. (1976). Management and outcome of pregnancies associated with the copper T intrauterine contraceptive device. *American Journal of Obstetrics and Gynecology*, **126**, 869−879.

Teper, S. (1978). Female sterilization in Aberdeen: preliminary findings. *Population Studies*, **32**, 549−566.

Teper, S. and Clarke, J. (1979). Female sterilization in Scotland (to be published).

Thomas, D.B. (1972). Relationship of oral contraception to cervical carcinogenesis. *Obstetrics and Gynecology*, **40**, 508−518.

Tietze, C. (1959). The clinical effectiveness of contraceptive methods. *American Journal of Obstetrics and Gynecology*, **78**, 650−656.

Tietze, C. (1978). Repeat abortions − why more? *Family Planning Perspectives* **10**, 286−288.

Tietze, C. (1979). The pill and mortality from cardiovascular disease: another look. *International Family Planning Perspectives*, **5**, 8−12.

Tietze, C., Bongaarts, J. and Schearer, B. (1976). Mortality associated with the control of fertility. *Family Planning Perspectives*, **8**, 6−14.

Tietze, C. and Jain, A.K. (1978). The mathematics of repeat abortion: explaining the increase. *Studies in Family Planning*, **9**, 294−299.

Tietze, C. and Lewit, S. (1968). Statistical evaluation of contraceptive methods: use-effectiveness and extended use-effectiveness. *Demography*, **5**, 931.

Tietze, C. and Lewit, S. (1970). Evaluation and intrauterine devices: ninth progress report on the Cooperative Statistical Program. *Studies in Family Planning*, **55**, 1−40.

Timonen, H. and Luukkainen, T. (1974). Immediate postabortion insertion of the Copper-T (TCu-200) with eighteen months follow-up. *Contraception*, **9**, 153−160.

U.S. Department of Health, Education and Welfare (1979). *Patterns of Aggregate and Individual Changes in Contraceptive Practice, United States, 1965−1975*. Analytical Studies, Series 3, No. 17. Washington, DC.

Vana, J., Murphy, G.P., Arnoff, B.L. and Baker, H.W. (1977). Study of association between liver tumours and oral contraceptive use. Unpublished, cited in *Population Reports* (1977).

Vaughan, B., Trussell, J., Menken, J. and Jones, E.F. (1977). Contraceptive failure among married women in the United States, 1970−1973. *Family Planning Perspectives*, **9**, 251−258.

Vessey, M.P. (1979). Oral contraception and neoplasia. *British Journal of Family Planning*, **4**, 65, 69−71.

Vessey, M.P., Doll, R. and Jones, K. (1975). Oral contraceptives and breast cancer: progress report of an epidemiological study, *Lancet*, **i**, 941−944.

Vessey, M.P., Doll, R., Johnson, B. and Peto, R. (1974). Outcome of pregnancy in women using an intrauterine device. *Lancet*, **i**, 495.

Vessey, M.P., Doll, R., Peto, R., Johnson, B. and Wiggins, P. (1976). A long-term follow-up study of women using different methods of contraception − an interim report. *Journal of Biosocial Science*, **8**, 373−427.

Vessey, M.P., McPherson, K. and Johnson, B. (1977). Mortality among women participating in the Oxford Family Planning Association contraceptive study. *Lancet*, **ii**, 731−733.

Vessey, M.P., Wright, N.H., McPherson, K. and Wiggins, P. (1978). Fertility after stopping different methods of contraception. *British Medical Journal*, **i**, 265−267.

Vessey, M.P., Doll, R., Jones, K., McPherson, K. and Yeates, D., (1979). An epidemiological study of oral contraceptives and breast cancer. *British Medical Journal*, i, 1757–1760.

Westoff, C.F. and Jones, E.F. (1977). Contraception and sterilization in the United States. *Family Planning Perspectives*, **9**, 153–157.

Weström, L. (1975). Effect of acute pelvic inflammatory disease on fertility. *American Journal of Obstetrics and Gynecology*, **121**, 707–713.

Weström, L., Bengtsson, L.P. and Mårdh, P.-A. (1976). The risk of pelvic inflammatory disease in women using intrauterine contraceptive devices as compared to non-users. *Lancet*, ii, 221–224.

Wilson, E. (1976). Use of long-acting depo progesterone in domiciliary family planning. *British Medical Journal*, ii, 1435–1437.

Winston, R.M.L. (1977). Why 103 women asked for reversal of sterilization. *British Medical Journal*, ii, 305–307.

World Health Organisation (1978). *Risk Approach for Maternal and Child Health Care:* Offset publication No. 39. Geneva: WHO.

World Health Organisation (1979a). Gestation, birth-weight, and spontaneous abortion in pregnancy after induced abortion. Report of collaborative study by WHO task force on sequelae of abortion. *Lancet*, i, 142–145.

World Health Organisation (1979b). Special programme of research, development and research training in human reproduction. An assessment of the Lippes Loop D and the Copper TC 220C. *Health Report Programme/79, Rev. 1.* Geneva: WHO.

Worth, A.J. and Boyes, D.A. (1972). A case control study into the possible effects of birth control pill on pre-clinical carcinoma of the cervix. *Journal of Obstetrics and Gynaecology of the British Commonwealth*, **79**, 673–679.

Ylikorkala, O. (1977). Ovarian cysts and hormonal contraception. *Lancet.* i, 1101–1102.

Causes and Treatment of Involuntary Childlessness — Recent Advances

M.C. MACNAUGHTON

University Department of Obstetrics and Gynaecology, Royal Maternity Hospital, Glasgow, Scotland

The incidence of involuntary infertility in the population is not known with accuracy. It is therefore only possible to make an indirect estimate of the figure and it probably nears 10 per cent (Cooke, 1977). About 10 per cent of couples in the UK remain childless, but this figure also contains a number of couples who have decided not to have children so that the proportion in which infertility is involuntary is not known. There are no data to distinguish between voluntary and involuntary infertility and most well-documented infertility studies are from infertility clinics where the data may be biased due to the particular interests of the person involved.

In certain areas of the world such as tropical Africa, there is a particularly high incidence of infertility, mainly due to tubal blockage resulting from pelvic inflammatory disease (Adadevoh, 1974). It is probable that in these countries the endocrine causes of infertility which are relatively more important in the UK are also present, but are overshadowed by the number due to tubal blockage.

In the main, the advances in the aetiology and treatment of infertility relate to the female but it seems probable that male factors contribute significantly in 35 to 40 per cent of infertile marriages (de Kretser, 1974). In recent years more knowledge has been gained, especially about the endocrine factors in the male resulting in infertility and here some success has been recorded.

Male Infertility

The failure of the male pituitary to secrete follicle stimulating hormone (FSH) and luteinizing hormone (LH) results in abnormal testicular function and infertility. In men with infertility, gonadotrophin deficiency accounts for less than 0·5 per cent of the causative factors. Correction of these deficiencies can result in successful spermatogenesis being restored, but careful evaluation is required to achieve this. In spite of the fact that gonadotrophin deficiency is a rare cause of male infertility, measurements of FSH, LH, prolactin and testosterone can be useful in the management of male infertility. FSH measurements are of most importance since there are relationships between FSH concentration and the state of the seminiferous epithelium. The higher the FSH concentration, the greater the damage to the epithelium. The epithelium presumably fails to produce adequate feedback to lower the FSH concentration (de Kretser *et al.*, 1974). The measurement of FSH may now be used instead of testicular biopsy as a measure of the state of the seminiferous epithelium in men with severe reduction of sperm count. In a man with azoospermia and a normal FSH concentration the epithelium will be normal. If the FSH is elevated the epithelium shows damage.

The modern investigation of the infertile male is more complex than before and involves thorough investigation by seminal analysis and endocrine evaluation. It is now important to locate the lesion responsible for infertility and institute logical treatment. This is now possible, owing particularly to the advances in knowledge of the physiology of reproduction in the male. A number of drugs are available today and their use should be determined after proper evaluation of the likely cause of the infertility.

Hormones have been used in the treatment of testicular disorders and the treatment has both been specific and non-specific. Although there are only a small number of patients with demonstrated gonadotrophin deficiency, treatment by replacement therapy is often successful in restoring the sperm count. Treatment has to be continued for up to 18 months. If treatment is performed in well-selected cases, such as men who have had hypophysectomy (Table I) or who have hypogonado-

Table I
Response to hMG/hCG treatment

	No. of patients	Instances of complete spermatogenesis
Patients after hypophysectomy	20	20
Patients with hypogonadotropic hypogonadism	33	27

Source: after Lunenfeld and Insler, 1978.

Table II
Effect of gonadotrophins on oligospermic men

No. of Patients	Improvement to moderate oligospermic	Fertility proven by pregnancy
275	76	20 (7%)

Source: after Lunenfeld and Insler, 1978.

trophic hypogonadism, the results are very good, but if gonadotrophins are used in unselected cases the results are poor (Table II).

Clomiphene has also been used to elevate gonadotrophin concentration and may be beneficial if the lesion has been diagnosed as one of feedback failure.

Androgens have frequently been used in the treatment of azoospermia or oligospermia on the basis that the hormone will suppress spermatogenesis and when treatment is stopped the sperm count will rebound to higher concentrations than in the pre-treatment phase. The results of this therapy have never been properly evaluated and proper trials are required.

While it is possible, therefore, to restore fertility in a number of infertile men, especially those with isolated gonadotrophin deficiency, the fact that there are so many different treatments (Table III) suggests that there is still much work to be done in this field. However, the growing knowledge of the physiology of reproduction has resulted in improvements and this should make the challenge easier to meet.

Table III
Therapeutic possibilities in male infertility

1. Gonadotrophins
2. Clomiphene
3. Gonadotrophin releasing hormone
4. Androgens
5. Antibiotics
6. Sperm vitalizing therapy
7. Corrective surgery
8. 'Split' intercourse
9. Therapeutic inseminations

Source: Lunenfeld and Insler, 1978.

In Vitro Fertilization and Embryo Transfer

One of the more dramatic advances of recent times in the treatment of infertility due to tubal blockage or absence of the fallopian tubes is the method of *in vitro* fertilization and embryo transfer. Very recently the first success was obtained in the field of human fertilization *in vitro*, when Steptoe and Edwards (1978) showed that this technique was applicable to the human. This work has been more fully described in a lecture by Steptoe and Edwards at the meeting of the Royal College of Obstetricians and Gynaecologists in January 1979. This team have established that *in vitro* fertilization and embryo transfer is a feasible approach to the treatment of infertility resulting from blockage or absence of the fallopian tubes.

Patients who have blocked or absent tubes but who have a normal ovary, normal tube, normal uterus and a normal husband are suitable for this technique. Firstly, a diagnostic laparoscopy is performed to assess the possibility of recovering an oocyte from the ovary. If the patient is thought to be suitable for this type of treatment pre-ovulatory eggs are aspirated from the ovary about four to six hours before ovulation, which has been induced by the injections of human chorionic gonadotrophin (hCG) 32 hours previously. It is possible to obtain an increased number of oocytes by stimulating follicular growth by treatment with human menopausal gonadotrophin (hMG) or clomiphene but it can also be done from normal follicles before spontaneous ovulation. *In vitro* fertilization is then performed in a laboratory and the resultant fertilized egg is then grown in culture and reimplanted into the uterus through the cervix.

When the series of experiments was reported at the Royal College of Obstetricians and Gynaecologists there had been 32 implantations of fertilized eggs and four pregnancies had resulted. In two of these a live child was delivered and in the other two, spontaneous abortion occurred at 10 and 20 weeks' gestation.

Another approach to this problem would be to recover several oocytes at a single laparotomy after stimulation of the ovaries, to store these at a low temperature either as oocytes or after fertilization and then to transfer them to the recipient in future normal cycles. Since abnormally high concentrations of steroid hormones result from gonadotrophin treatment the chances of implantation and normal pregnancy are likely to be greater if the *in vitro* fertilized embryo can be stored and returned to the mother's uterus when normal cycles have been resumed (Willadsen, 1977). This work of Steptoe and Edwards has established conclusively that *in vitro* fertilization and embryo transfer is a feasible approach to the treatment of infertility resulting from blockage or absence of the tubes. The demand for this type of treatment is likely to increase, particularly in countries where tubal blockages are a major cause of infertility. Further research is required and there is a great need for a meticulous scientific appraisal of the risks, benefits and causes of failure of the whole procedure. Research with human oocyte and sperm involve deep ethical problems and these also have to be considered. In the setting of treatment, collaboration between skilled clinicians and laboratory workers is essential if progress is to be made. The technique will be expensive in human resources and this type of treatment should probably be conducted in a small number of centres where the expertise is available.

Female Infertility

It is really the improvement in understanding of the endocrine control of the ovarian cycle that has made the rational treatment of endocrine causes of female infertility possible in recent years.

The female menstrual cycle is under the over-all control of the higher centres, and sensory stimuli from the external environment such as stress, visual and olfactory stimuli cause release of neurotransmitters such as catecholamines, indolamines and cholinergic agents. These act on the hypothalamus to regulate the control of gonadotrophic releasing hormones which in turn cause the release of gonadotrophins (FSH and LH). These act on the ovary, which is stimulated to produce the ovarian steroid hormones, mainly oestrogen and progesterone, which act on the endometrium of the uterus. Oestradiol is the most important hormone regulating the secretion of pituitary gonadotrophin. It has a double action. It acts by a negative feedback mechanism at the hypothalamic and pituitary levels to inhibit the secretion of gonadotrophins, whereas by a positive feedback mechanism it is also responsible at mid-cycle for stimulating a discharge of LH and FSH resulting in ovulation in the mature follicle. The positive feedback of oestrogen is both dose and time dependent and in normal women makes sure that only the mature graafian follicle induces the pre-ovulatory LH discharge. Any disruption in the interaction between the various components of the hypothalamo−pituitary−ovarian axis may lead to anovulation, which is one of the main causes of infertility in the human female (Baird *et al.*, 1976).

Diagnostic Tests

In recent years it has become clearer what diagnostic tests are required in the investigation of women complaining of infertility. First, it is essential in all women complaining of infertility to take a comprehensive history and make a thorough physical examination. Laparoscopy should be performed to visualize the pelvic organs and assess their normality or otherwise. At the same time with hydro-tubation the patency of the fallopian tubes is assessed. This method of assessing the patency is an improvement over the previously used method of insufflation with gas. Endometrial biopsy in the luteal phase of the cycle is essential, and finally hormonal assays will be required but for which hormone will depend to some extent on the individual case and facilities that are present.

It is the development of accurate assays of a variety of hormones in plasma by radioimmunoassay that has revolutionized the diagnosis of female infertility. The very low levels of these hormones which regulate the menstrual cycle can now be accurately measured in small quantities of blood so that by taking samples daily, or in some cases even more frequently, throughout the cycle a much more accurate assessment of the activity of the different organs can be obtained and the different levels can be correlated in the same patient. In this way, variations from the normal can be detected and attempts made to correct the abnormality. This has been a major advance in recent years. In cases of amenorrhoea and oligomenorrhoea, knowledge of the blood levels of prolactin, FSH, LH and thyroxin is essential. The assessment of the spontaneous ovarian activity by weekly (or more frequent) measurements of oestradiol and progesterone or their urinary conjugates should be carried out. As an alternative or an adjuvant in women with amenorrhoea or oligomenorrhoea, the uterine response to exogenous progesterone should be ascertained. Withdrawal of progesterone will only cause bleeding if the uterus has already been primed with oestrogen so that a positive progesterone withdrawal test indicates some spontaneous ovarian activity (Kletzky et al., 1975).

Lastly, X-ray examination of the pituitary fossa for pituitary tumour is necessary. If the skull X-ray is abnormal, then full radiological examination with tomography is essential to determine the extent of the abnormality.

In the UK, endocrine conditions are an important cause of infertility and in this area great advances have been made in the last 10–15 years. The endocrine conditions can be divided into two main types: those in which ovulation does not occur — anovulatory infertility — and those in which ovulation occurs but is inadequate.

Anovulatory Infertility

It is possible by the tests described to divide patients with anovulatory infertility into two groups: those who suffer from ovarian failure and those with gonadotrophin failure.

Patients with ovarian failure have ovaries which do not contain any oocytes, so that the level of gonadotrophins is raised markedly (Goldenberg et al., 1973). It is also possible for ovarian failure to be primary, and this is found in patients with genetic disorders such as Turner's syndrome where the chromosome constitution is abnormal. It may also occur after a period of normal menstruation, and in such patients this also can be due to a chromosomal abnormality since it has been shown that many patients with chromosome abnormalities have a reduced number of oocytes. Their ovarian function is present for some years until, as it were, the supply is used up. The cause of ovarian failure is not known although an autoimmune basis has been suggested. There is no treatment available for this condition.

Patients with gonadotrophin failure have a more hopeful prognosis. Most of the patients with this abnormality have basal levels of gonadotrophins within the normal range but it is possible by measuring prolactin, FSH, LH and oestradiol concentration, to divide them into four groups — those with hyperprolactinaemia and those with normal levels of prolactin; those with polycystic ovarian disease and those with thyroid disease.

About 20 per cent of women with secondary amenorrhoea have levels of prolactin above normal and some have in addition galactorrhoea (Jacobs, 1976). One-third of women with hyperprolactinaemia have pituitary tumours, the majority of which are chromophobe adenomas.

If a tumour is present it can be removed surgically although this may result in permanent hypopituitarism in a small number of women. Since the pituitary enlarges in pregnancy, if a tumour is present there is a risk of its further growth during pregnancy and this may cause adverse symptoms due to pressure on the surrounding structures (Gemzell, 1965). The best compromise is probably to treat the bigger tumours by surgery and those that are small by chemical means. This means the use of the dopamine agonist bromocriptine (Parlodel). When this is given, very close observation of the patient is essential in case there should be symptoms of pituitary enlargement.

When hyperprolactinaemia is present in the absence of a tumour, the concentrations of FSH and LH present are related to a lower concentration of oestrogen than normal and Van Look et al. (1977) have suggested that prolactin may directly inhibit follicular development or ovarian secretion. In hyperprolactinaemia without tumour, treatment is with bromocriptine. This is very effective and fertility rates are good (Thorner et al., 1975).

The women with normal prolactin levels can be divided into those with normal gonadotrophin levels and those with low gonadotrophins. The former group usually have normal follicular levels of oestrogen and bleed after the withdrawal of exogenous progesterone. It is not clear why these women are abnormal, but it has been suggested that the negative feedback mechanism is abnormal and that minimal quantities of oestrogen inhibit the secretion of pituitary gonadotrophins (Baird, 1979).

These patients can be treated very successfully by anti-oestrogenic drugs such as clomiphene or tamoxifen. Ovulation rates following the use of clomiphene vary from 50 per cent (Pildes, 1965) to 96 per cent (Kistner, 1965). However, in spite of the high rates of ovulation that are obtained, pregnancy rates are rather low even though there is good biochemical evidence of ovulation. It has been suggested that this may be due to the effect of the anti-oestrogen on the cervical mucus which, as a result, remains hostile to the passage of sperm. These women have been treated in addition by giving ethanol oestradiol from days 5−10 of the cycle (Insler et al., 1973). Although successful results have been claimed, further controlled work is necessary on this subject before this therapy is established.

In patients with low gonadotrophins there is failure of the hypothalamus or anterior pituitary. Low levels of oestrogen are present and therefore the uterus does not bleed on the withdrawal of exogenous progesterone. These patients can be treated successfully by gonadotrophin therapy. In the patients who also have severe weight loss, as is found in anorexia nervosa, psychiatric therapy and treatment to restore a normal body weight will usually result in normal ovarian activity. In some of these women, however, exogenous gonadotrophins are necessary to induce ovulation. This therapy has been in use now for over 20 years and is well established. It involves stimulating follicular development by serial injections of human menopausal gonadotrophin (hMG). When satisfactory development has been achieved, as measured usually by daily oestrogen levels in plasma or urine, ovulation is induced by chorionic gonadotrophin. In properly selected and monitored patients, between 60 and 75 per cent will become pregnant and it has been concluded that, as far as this type of anovulatory infertility is concerned, it is a curable disease (Lunenfeld and Insler, 1978).

A new development in the monitoring of follicular growth during induction of ovulation is the use of ultrasound. Serial measurements of individual follicles of at least 10 mm in size can be made. It has been shown that there is a close correlation between follicular size as measured by ultrasound and the level of oestradiol in the serum (Hackeloer *et al.*, 1979). It is now likely that in future the timing of ovulation will be measured by this method.

In some patients with anovulatory infertility clinical features are present which suggest a polycystic ovary syndrome. These are hirsutism, obesity and a disturbance in menstrual rhythm. The ovaries in these women are enlarged and sclerocystic and ovulation does not occur. Histological examination of these ovaries shows numerous follicular cysts under the capsule of the ovary, and corpora atretica are also present. The theca interna is often hyperplastic and may be luteinized. The stroma does not usually show much change but hyperplasia and luteinization have been reported. Levels of LH are elevated in these patients and this, presumably, is responsible for the luteinization. These ovaries secrete very little oestrogen and a large amount of androgen. Although it has been suggested that this abnormality in steroid secretion is due to a genetic deficiency in the ability to aromatize androgens to oestrogens, it is possible to induce follicular growth in these women with exogenous gonadotrophins or clomiphene. This suggests that the ovarian defect may be secondary to an inappropriate stimulation by gonadotrophins and, although the pattern of the secretion of LH and FSH is abnormal, there does not seem to be an intrinsic deficiency in the hypothalamo—pituitary feedback mechanism. In patients with poly-cystic ovarian disease the amount of oestrogen secreted by the ovary is small. Most of the oestrogen is produced by the extra-glandular conversion of androgen in the liver and fat (Siiteri and MacDonald, 1973). As a result, the hypothalamo—pituitary system is exposed to oestrogen produced from outside the ovary and the ovarian cycle stops.

Clomiphene is effective in the treatment of polycystic ovarian disease and increases the secretion of endogenous FSH. The other successful treatment is wedge resection of the ovaries. This results in the restoration of ovulation in 70—80 per cent of cases and Dorfman (1963) described a fall in plasma androgen after wedge resection, perhaps because of a reduction of the amount of precursor androgen available for extra-glandular conversion with a subsequent reduction of oestrogen. The hypothalamo—pituitary system would then not be suppressed (Baird,

1979). The aetiology of the condition is unknown but it has been suggested that a temporary period of adrenal hyperactivity at the menarche or hyperactivity due to stress may precipitate the anovulatory polycystic ovary in susceptible subjects (Yen, 1978).

Thyroid disease can also result in ovarian failure. The synthesis of sex hormone binding globulin (SHBG) is stimulated by thyroid hormones. In hyperthyroidism there is an increase in the amount of oestrogen bound to SHBG and there is also an increase in the extra-glandular conversion of androgens to oestrogens so that a situation arises very like that in the polycystic ovary syndrome. Hypothyroidism results in an increase of the metabolic clearance rate of both testosterone and oestradiol because of increased binding. Treatment in the case of hyperthyroidism is by anti-thyroid drugs or surgery and by thyroxin in the case of hypothyroidism.

Inadequate Ovulation

The last group of endocrine patients to be discussed are perhaps the most difficult to understand. Many women who are infertile after the usual investigations seem to be normal and to have normal menstrual cycles with apparent ovulation. It is difficult to put these patients into categories because many of them seem to be different from each other. There are patients who have apparently normal menstrual cycles, there is no abnormality seen on laparoscopic examination, the fallopian tubes are patent and the husbands are normal. The only abnormality is an inability to conceive after trying to do so for a minimum of three years. These patients have been studied by taking daily samples of blood during a menstrual cycle and assaying FSH, LH, prolactin, oestradiol and progesterone. In a former study we suggested that the defect in these women was concerned with ovulation of a poorly grown follicle (Dodson et al., 1975a) and this work was confirmed by Cooke (1977).

In these patients the levels of FSH were basically normal throughout the cycle although the levels at the beginning and end of the cycle were much more variable than in normal women. Levels of LH were high normal, particularly in the follicular phase. The levels of prolactin were also very variable and the mean data show that the levels were in the upper range for our normal 95 per cent confidence limits. The levels of oestradiol 17 B and progesterone confirmed, particularly in some individual patients, our previous findings that the pre-ovulatory rise in oestradiol was less than that observed in the normal cycle and that the luteal levels of oestradiol and progesterone were also reduced (Coutts *et al.*, 1979).

Grouping these patients together obscured some of the individual abnormalities, and in a group like this with a probably mixed aetiology, the individual patient can act as her own control.

Since high prolactin levels had been observed in the patients as a group, individual prolactin results have been examined. As a result, a group has been identified and the abnormality called transient hyperprolactinaemia (T↑PRL). This has been defined as occurring in any cycle where one or more but not all samples show prolactin levels above the 95 per cent confidence limits for the normal data. Statistically, 5 per cent of values should fall outside these limits (2·5 per cent above and below). Therefore in a 28-day menstrual cycle less than one sample would be expected to lie above these limits (Coutts *et al.*, 1979).

Although one sample above the level was taken for the definition of transient hyperprolactinaemia, very few patients had only one or two raised prolactin levels. The number of days on which prolactin values were elevated range from 1−17, the mean being 6 days ± 4 days. In 30 infertile patients in the study, 20 of them had transient hyperprolactinaemia. Even if the definition was changed to include only patients who had three or more raised prolactin levels the incidence is still more than 50 per cent.

To understand better the possible effects of these prolactin levels in both stages of the cycle, the correlations between prolactin levels and oestradiol and progesterone levels at different stages of the cycle were studied. It was found that there was a significant negative correlation between the mean mid-cycle (day −2 to day +2, on either side of the mid-cycle LH peak) level and the total luteal level of oestradiol. The relationship was even more marked when only late luteal (day +9 to the onset of menstruation) was compared to mid-cycle prolactin. Presumably high prolactin levels at the time of formation of the luteotrophic complex would interfere with its formation. As far as progesterone is concerned, again the only significant one relates mid-cycle prolactin levels to luteal progesterone levels. The luteal levels of progesterone in the hyperprolactinaemic group were significantly lower than those in normal prolactin women. These findings are consistent with the *in vitro* studies of McNatty *et al.* (1974) who observed that above a certain level prolactin had a deleterious effect on the production of progesterone by cultured isolated human granulosa cells. It seems likely, therefore, that elevated prolactin levels at the time of the formation of the luteotrophic complex interferes with the life-span of the corpus luteum and results in a reduction, particularly by the late corpus luteum, in the synthesis of ovarian steroids.

Three main groups of luteal phase abnormality have been observed in these infertile patients. In the first group there was a short luteal phase, and all patients had transient hyperprolactinaemia; Sherman and Korenman (1974) defined a short luteal phase as one where the luteal phase lasted 11 days or less. A second group had a poor surge of progesterone, i.e. where the luteal production of progesterone does not accelerate as fast as it does in normal cycles. There is also a sub-group of patients within this group with poor progesterone surge and associated elevated LH levels. Thirdly, there is a group where luteal progesterone and oestradiol were both low.

Most patient groups had a proportion with transient hyperprolactinaemia but it was only in the patients with the short luteal phase that prolactin levels were raised in all cases. This group is of particular interest since there is a significant correlation between the mean mid-cycle prolactin level and the length of the luteal phase. In the light of the effects of mid-cycle prolactin on late luteal steroidogenesis already mentioned, it seems likely that the elevated mid-cycle prolactin is responsible for the short luteal phase. Support for these conclusions can also be drawn from reports that women with amenorrhoea, as a result of very elevated prolactin levels, having treatment with bromocriptine experience short luteal phases before their cycle returns to normal (Del Pozo *et al.*, 1976).

Treatment of Inadequate Ovulation

The treatment varies with the possible cause as determined by the hormone profile. Three main drugs have been used: (1) clomiphene; (2) human menopausal gonadotrophin (Pergonal); and (3) bromocriptine (Parlodel).

1. *Clomiphene.* This was the drug used initially in this work. The findings have already been reported (Dodson, *et al.*, 1975a, b) and will only be summarized here. The main finding in this group of patients, which numbered 12, was a low level of FSH in the late luteal phase. Oestradiol levels were low in the follicular and early luteal phase with a 'stagger' to the luteal peak. Progesterone levels showed a slow rise to a late peak. These patients were treated with 50 mg clomiphene from day 1−5 of the cycle. The treatment resulted in a marked increase in plasma FSH, oestradiol and

progesterone levels and showed that follicle stimulation had occurred with a resultant improvement in luteal function. This response to treatment demonstrated the interrelationship between follicular growth and luteal function. However, the pregnancy rate was disappointing, only one pregnancy resulting. It is possible that this is due to the anti-oestrogenic effect of clomiphene on the cervical mucus already mentioned.

2. *Human menopausal gonadotrophin (hMG–Pergonal)*. Since 1958 hMG has been used to produce ovulation in amenorrhoeic women (Gemzell *et al.*, 1958). In view of the deficiency of the follicular phase, in many of these women it was considered rational to give hMG to stimulate the follicle and therefore the corpus luteum. hMG was given to 21 patients. The response varied from anovulation to pregnancy. Fourteen patients had transient hyperprolactinaemia, seven were normal prolactinaemic; five women became pregnant and all were in the poor progesterone surge group. hMG would therefore seem the most suitable treatment for this type of patient (Macnaughton *et al.*, 1979).

3. *Bromocriptine (Parlodel)*. Prolactin has been shown to be important in corpus luteum function in the human (Delvoye *et al.*, 1974) and it has been shown that the elevated levels may cause a short luteal phase. Prolactin, therefore has an effect on the luteotrophic complex (Del Pozo *et al.*, 1976). A moderate

Table IV
Poor progesterone surge patients: effect of bromocriptine (2·5 mg daily)

Hormone	Follicular phase (1st day to -2)	Mid-cycle (days -2 to $+2$)	Luteal phase (days $+3$ to end)
FSH (mIU/ml ± s.d.)			
Pre-treatment	$5·0 \pm 0·9$	$7·4 \pm 4·4$	$3·4 \pm 1·4$
Bromocriptine	$3·9 \pm 0·6$	$5·8 \pm 2·3$	$2·2 \pm 0·8$
p	$< 0·025^a$	$< 0·15$	$< 0·01^a$
LH (mIU/ml ± s.d.)			
Pre-treatment	$5·8 \pm 0·53$	$15·2 \pm 9·0$	$5·6 \pm 2·0$
Bromocriptine	$4·5 \pm 0·4$	$12·3 \pm 7·5$	$3·7 \pm 1·3$
p	$< 0·001^a$	$< 0·1$	$< 0·005^a$

[a] Significant.

increase in the prolactin level has been reported in patients with luteal insufficiency (Seppälä *et al.*, 1976). From our studies in patients with a poor progesterone surge, bromocriptine causes a fall in both FSH and LH and luteal phases of the cycle (Table IV).

It is known that dopamine is associated with the control of the tonic levels of LH and it is evident from the results in Table IV

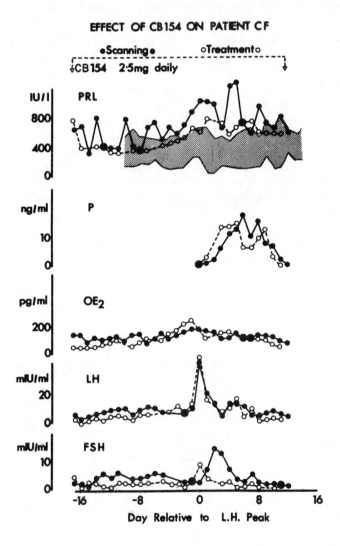

FIG. 1. Effect of bromocriptine (CB154) on the short luteal phase. No change owing to failure to reduce prolactin level.

that the levels are lowered by bromocriptine especially in the follicular and luteal phases. FSH seems also to be reduced at these times. This reduction of FSH levels in the follicular phase may mean that bromocriptine is having two opposite treatment effects. Where it is acting to reduce the level of prolactin it may improve the function of the corpus luteum, but it may at the same time lower FSH levels in the follicular phase and reduce the

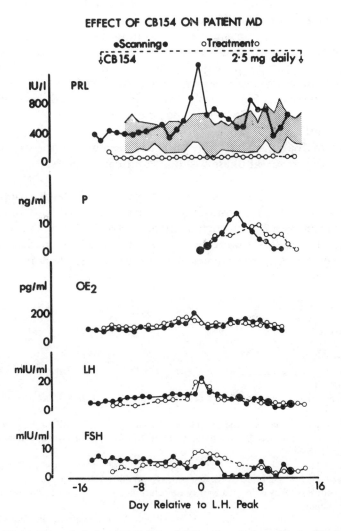

FIG. 2. Effect of bromocriptine (CB154) on the short luteal phase. Normal luteal length achieved after lowering of prolactin level.

stimulus to follicular growth. This in turn may result in deficient follicular growth and secondary corpus luteum abnormality. It is suggested, therefore, that in certain women with transient hyper-prolactinaemia bromocriptine may be best given at mid-cycle for 3 days on each side of the luteal peak. In addition, in some patients, it may be necessary to give a combination of hMG on days 1, 3, and 5 of the cycle as well as the mid-cycle bromo-criptine. There are different possible combinations of these two drugs and further work is required in this field.

Bromocriptine may be successful in the treatment of the short luteal phase and Figs 1 and 2 show the results in two such patients. In the patient in Fig. 1, bromocriptine did not reduce the prolactin level sufficiently and the short luteal phase continued. In the case in Fig. 2, prolactin levels were lowered throughout the cycle on bromocriptine and the luteal phase was normal in length.

hCG and progesterone have also been used in the treatment of deficient luteal phase without significant success.

There are, therefore, many types of treatment of infertility depending on the cause. Much painstaking research is required to delineate the different problems and then controlled trials will be necessary to evaluate the results. However, much progress has been made in the last 15 – 20 years and it is to be hoped that in the next decade similar progress will continue.

References

Adadevoh, B.K. (Editor) (1974). *Subfertility and Infertility in Africa.* Ibadan, Nigeria: Caxton Press.

Baird, D.T. (1979). Endocrinology of female infertility. *British Medical Bulletin,* **35,** 193–198.

Baird, D.T., Van Look, F.P.A. and Hunter, W.M. (1976). Classification of abnormal patterns of gonadotrophin release in women. *Clinics in Obstetrics and Gynaecology,* **3,** 505–513.

Cooke, I.D. (1977). The natural history and major causes of infertility. In *Regulation of Human Fertility,* edited by E. Diczfalusy, pp. 88–110. Proceedings of a WHO Symposium on Advances in Fertility Regulation, Moscow, 16–19 November 1976. Copenhagen: Scriptor.

Coutts, J.R.T., Fleming, R., Carswell, W., Black, W.P., England, P., Craig, A. and Macnaughton, M.C. (1979). The defective luteal phase. In *Advances in Gynae-cological Endocrinology,* edited by H.S. Jacobs, pp. 65–91. Proceedings of the Sixth

Study Group of the Royal College of Obstetricians and Gynaecologists. London.
de Kretser, D.M. (1974). The management of the infertile male. *Clinics in Obstetrics and Gynaecology*, 1, 409–427.
de Kretser, D.M., Berger, H.G. and Hudson, B. (1974). Diagnostic aspects of male infertility. In *Proceedings of Serona Symposium on Male Reproduction*, edited by R.E Mancini and L. Martini. New York and London: Academic Press.
Del Pozo, E., Wyss, H., Lancranjan, I., Obolensky, W. and Jarga, L. (1976). Prolactin induced luteal insufficiency and its treatment with bromocriptine: preliminary results. In *Ovulation in the Human*, edited by P.G. Crosignani and D.R. Mishell, pp. 297–299. London: Academic Press.
Delvoye, P., Taubert, H.D., Jurgensen, D., L'Hermite, M., Delogne, J. and Robyn, C. (1974). Influence of circulating prolactin increased by a psychotrophic drug on gonadotrophin and progesterone secretion. *Acta Endocrinologica (Copenhagen) Supplement*, 184, 110.
Dodson, K.S., Macnaughton, M.C. and Coutts, J.R.T. (1975a). Infertility in women with apparently normal ovulatory cycles. 1. Comparison of their plasma sex steroid and gonadotrophin profiles with those in the normal cycle. *British Journal of Obstetrics and Gynaecology*, 82, 615–624.
Dodson, K.S., Macnaughton, M.C. and Coutts, J.R.T. (1975b). Infertility in women with apparently ovulatory cycles. 2. The effects of clomiphene treatment on the profiles of gonadotrophin and sex steroid hormones in peripheral plasma. *British Journal of Obstetrics and Gynaecology*, 82, 625–633.
Dorfman, R.I. (1963). Steroid hormones in gynaecology. *Obstetric and Gynecological Survey*, 18, 65–116.
Gemzell, C.A. (1965). Induction of ovulation with human gonadotrophins. *Recent Progress in Hormone Research*, 21, 179–198.
Gemzell, C.A., Diczfalusy, E. and Tillinger, K.G. (1958). Clinical effect of human pituitary follicle stimulating hormone (FSH). *Journal of Clinical Endocrinology*, 18, 138–148.
Goldenberg, R.L., Grodin, J.M., Rodbard, D. and Ross, G.T. (1973). Gonadotrophins in women with amenorrhoea. *American Journal of Obstetrics and Gynecology*, 116, 1003–1009.
Hackeloer, B.J., Fleming, R., Robinson, H.P., Adam, A.H. and Coutts, J.R.T. (1979). Correlation of ultrasonic and endocrinological assessment of human follicular development. *American Journal of Obstetrics and Gynecology*, 135, 122–128.
Insler, V., Zakut, H. and Serr, D.M. (1973). Cycle pattern and pregnancy rate following combined clomiphene-estrogen therapy. *Obstetrics and Gynecology*, 41, 602–607.
Jacobs, H.S. (1976). Failure of components of the negative feedback system. *Clinical Obstetrics and Gynecology*, 3, 515–534.
Kistner, R.W. (1965). Further observation on the effects of clomiphene citrate in anovulatory females. *American Journal of Obstetrics and Gynecology*, 92, 380–411.
Kletzky, O.A., Davajan, V., Jankamura, R.M., Thorneycroft, I.H. and Mishell, D.R. (1975). Clinical categorization of patients with secondary amenorrhoea using progesterone induced uterine bleeding and measurement of serum gonadotrophin levels. *American Journal of Obstetrics and Gynecology*, 121, 695–703.
Lunenfeld, B. and Insler, V. (1978). *Diagnosis and Treatment of Functional Infertility*. Berlin: Grosse-Verlag.
McNatty, K.P., Sawers, R.S. and McNeilly, A.S. (1974). A possible role for prolactin in the control of steroid secretion by the human graafian follicle. *Nature*, 250, 653–655.

Macnaughton, M.C., Fleming, R., Carswell, W., Black, W.P., England, P., Craig, A. and Coutts, J.R.T. (1979). Treatment of the defective luteal phase. In *Advances in Gynaecological Endocrinology*, edited by H.S. Jacobs, pp. 92–101. Proceedings of the Sixth Study Group of the Royal College of Obstetricians and Gynaecologists. London: Royal College of Obstetricians and Gynaecologists.

Pildes, R.B. (1965). Induction of ovulation with clomiphene. *American Journal of Obstetrics and Gynecology*, 91, 466–479.

Seppälä, M., Hirvonen, E., and Ranta, T. (1976). Bromocriptine treatment of secondary amenorrhoea. *Lancet*, i, 1154–1156.

Sherman, B.M. and Korenman, S.G. (1974). Measurement of plasma, LH, FSH, oestradiol and progesterone. In Disorders of the human menstrual cycle: the short luteal phase. *Journal of Clinical Endocrinology and Metabolism*, 38, 89.

Siiteri, P.K. and MacDonald, P.C. (1973). Role of extra glandular estrogen in human endocrinology. In *Handbook of Physiology*, Section 7, *Endocrinology*, Volume 2. *Female Reproductive System*, Part 1, edited by R.O. Greep, pp. 615–629. Washington, DC: American Physiological Society.

Steptoe, P.C. and Edwards, R.G. (1978). Birth after the reimplantation of a human embryo. *Lancet*, ii, 366.

Thorner, M.O., Besser, G.M., Jones, A., Dacie, J. and Jones, A.E. (1975). Bromocriptine treatment of female infertility: report of thirteen pregnancies. *British Medical Journal*, iv, 694–697.

Van Look, P.F.A., McNeilly, A.S., Hunter, W.M. and Baird, D.T. (1977). The role of prolactin in secondary amenorrhoea. In *Prolactin and Human Reproduction*, edited by P.G. Crosignani and C. Robyn, pp. 217–224. Proceedings of the Serono Symposia Volume 11. London: Academic Press.

Willadsen, S.M. (1977). In *The Freezing of Mammalian Embryos*, pp. 175–189. CIBA Foundation Symposium 52 (New Series). Amsterdam: Elsevier, Excerpta Medica; London and New York: Associated Scientific Publishers.

Yen, S.S.C. (1978). In *Reproductive Endocrinology: Physiology, Pathophysiology and Clinical Management*, edited by S.S.C. Yen and R.B. Jaffe, pp. 297–323. Philadelphia and London: W.B. Saunders.

Avoiding Serious Birth Defects by Prenatal Diagnosis: Current Effects on Birth Incidence

M.A. FERGUSON–SMITH

Department of Medical Genetics, Royal Hospital for Sick Children, Yorkhill, Glasgow, Scotland

One of the purposes of the 1967 Abortion Act was to provide couples at substantial risk of having a seriously handicapped child the option of having the pregnancy terminated. As a decision on termination is much more acceptable if based on the certain knowledge rather than a statistical risk that the foetus is affected, there developed a demand for prenatal diagnostic tests. Prior to 1967 few such tests were available, the foetal sexing procedure for use in X-linked disorders being a notable exception (Riis and Fuchs, 1960). In fact, at the first Eugenics Society Symposium in 1964, the writer is recorded as expressing the view that it was doubtful if foetal chromosome analysis from embryonic cell cultures could be completed early enough in pregnancy to make therapeutic abortion possible (Ferguson-Smith, 1965). Thankfully, this prediction proved entirely false and two years later Steele and Breg (1966) published the first account of successful foetal chromosome analysis from amniotic fluid cell culture obtained by amniocentesis at 16 weeks' gestation. Shortly after, foetal chromosome aberrations were detected by this method. The ability to grow amniotic fluid cells in culture was soon exploited for the prenatal diagnosis of biochemical defects expressed in amniotic cells, and there are now over sixty inborn errors of metabolism which can be satisfactorily diagnosed *in utero* from such cultures. There have been added to the growing list of diagnosable foetal abnormalities over the past ten years major malformations of the central nervous system including spina bifida, sickle cell disease and the thalassaemias, exomphalos, congenital nephrosis, renal agenesis, polycystic kidneys, severe chondrodystrophies, microencephaly, haemophilia, myotonic dystrophy, congenital adrenal hyperplasia and many more (see, for example, Murken *et al.*, 1979). Prenatal diagnosis has become one of the major service commitments of Departments of Medical

Genetics. It has enlarged the scope and increased the value of genetic counselling and it is no exaggeration to say that it is the most effective measure currently available for the reduction of serious birth defects. It is therefore appropriate at this Symposium to examine the effects of the introduction of prenatal diagnosis on the prevalence of some of the conditions for which it has been used.

Chromosome Aberrations

It is widely recognized that the birth incidence of Down's syndrome, other autosomal trisomies and certain sex chromosome aberrations (XXX,XXY) increases with advancing maternal age. A recent analysis of 16 273 pregnancies collected from European Centres in women aged 35 years and over who had amniocentesis because of their age (Ferguson-Smith, 1979) shows that the incidence of trisomy 21 is 0·84 per cent in the maternal age group 35 − 39 years; if all chromosome aberrations are included the percentage of affected foetuses rises to 1·4 per cent. In the maternal age group 40 − 45 years, the frequencies have increased to 4·9 per cent and 8·2 per cent respectively (Table I). The figures for Down's syndrome are some 33 per cent higher than those obtained in less recent studies of the newborn and it is suggested that the discrepancy is explained in part by the loss of affected foetuses by abortion and stillbirth, and partly by a recent apparent increase in the birth incidence of Down's syndrome in the maternal age group 35 − 39 years (Evans et al., 1978). At any rate, it has been suggested that a maternal age of 35 years is an appropriate age to recommend screening by amniocentesis for foetal chromosome aberrations. One study estimates that the economic costs of providing prenatal diagnosis would be balanced by savings in health service resources used in the provision of care for surviving infants if mothers 35 years and over were tested (Hagard and Carter, 1976). This policy would be expected to reduce the number of births of Down's syndrome children by about 37 per cent.

Although maternal age of over 35 years is currently the most common indication for prenatal diagnosis, it appears that the proportion of total pregnancies being tested in such mothers is disappointingly small. For example, in a survey conducted by the Clinical Genetics Society (CGS) in 1976 (Ferguson-Smith et al., 1978a), it is estimated that less than 6 per cent of pregnant women aged 35 years and over had prenatal diagnosis. In that year, 71 (2·5 per cent) of 2837 pregnancies tested for this indication were found to be chromosomally abnormal: 33 had trisomic Down's syndrome. As a rough approximation, it appeared that prenatal

Table 1

Maternal age-specific risks (%) for all chromosome aberrations from Munich prenatal diagnosis data

Maternal age	Number of pregnancies	Trisomy-21	Other autosomal	XXY and XXX	Other sex chromosomal	Total abnormality rate (%)
35–39	8 742	0·86	0·25	0·19	0·08	1·38
40–44	7 011	2·04	0·88	0·51	0·06	3·49
45–49	518	5·60	1·39	1·18	–	8·17
35–49	16 273	1·52	0·58	0·37	0·06	2·47

diagnosis had reduced the birth incidence of Down's syndrome in 1976 by only 3 per cent. Assuming that a reduction of 37 per cent is theoretically possible if all women aged 35 and over had amniocentesis, this must be considered a disappointing result.

The most important factor responsible for this poor result appears to be the lack of provision of appropriate facilities for prenatal diagnosis. One large Regional Health Authority could provide no facilities in 1976 and nine others tested less than 1 per cent of all pregnancies, although facilities for testing 5–8 per cent of pregnancies would seem a reasonable requirement. Other contributory factors appear to be inadequate publicity and a failure of a large proportion of pregnant women to attend for antenatal care early enough. Older mothers with large families to care for often seem more reluctant than younger mothers to come to the clinic. Some obstetricians do not regard the risks of foetal chromosome aberration to be sufficiently high to justify risking the complications of amniocentesis, and others do not recommend the procedure unless the mother is over 40 years. Medical practitioners reluctant to advise their patients adequately on such matters, or to refer them for appropriate counselling, should take note of the legal implications, for it is understood that failure to advise about the availability of amniocentesis has already been the subject of legal proceedings in North America.

In some regions there is evidence that more mothers are coming forward to be tested than in 1976. In one report (Alberman et al., 1979) the proportion of pregnant women coming to be tested in the 40 years and over group had increased from 23 per cent in 1976 to 48 per cent in 1977. In our own local maternity hospital, where prenatal diagnosis has been available for ten years, the proportion of pregnant women 40 years and over who have prenatal diagnosis has remained virtually unchanged at between 50 and 55 per cent during the past three years. The proportion is even more disturbing when one takes the West of Scotland (with 36 000 deliveries per annum) as a whole, as the proportion of women in this age group tested has remained at 26 per cent for the past two years. It seems that the amniocentesis rate is unlikely to improve much unless some satisfactory means is found to persuade these women to attend earlier. Perhaps the French system of linking maternity benefits to early attendance for antenatal care should be considered for the United Kingdom.

Anencephaly and Spina Bifida

Since 1972, when it was first recognized that amniotic alphafoetoprotein

(AFP) levels could be used for the prenatal diagnosis of open neural tube defects (Brock and Sutcliffe, 1972), the risk of spina bifida has been one of the commonest indications for prenatal diagnosis. It had long been known that a woman with a history of one affected child with either anencephaly or spina bifida had a 1 in 20 risk of recurrence in each subsequent pregnancy. This risk frequently discouraged young couples from starting another pregnancy. The advent of the amniotic AFP test meant that these couples now had the opportunity of trying for a healthy child.

By 1976 the risk of recurrence of an open neural tube defect was the single commonest indication for prenatal diagnosis in the United Kingdom. The CGS Survey found that 1976 pregnancies had been tested that year and that 50 pregnancies (2·5 per cent) were affected. In high risk regions, like the West of Scotland, where neural tube defects occur in approximately six per 1000 births, a higher percentage of affected foetuses are found. Thus in 947 pregnancies tested for this indication up to the end of 1978, 4·4 per cent were abnormal; 34 open defects were detected and terminated and 8 closed defects continued to delivery.

It has been shown that in large series approximately 5 per cent of index patients with neural tube defects have had a previously affected sibling (Carter and Evans, 1979). A reduction of less than 5 per cent in the birth incidence of neural tube defects is therefore to be expected if all women with a previous history had prenatal diagnosis in a subsequent pregnancy. As it is likely that less than 25 per cent of women in this category undergo prenatal diagnosis, there would seem to be little opportunity for a major reduction in birth prevalence by this means. Fortunately, it has been discovered that in a large proportion of open neural tube defects there is an elevation of AFP levels in maternal serum. A UK Collaborative Study on maternal serum AFP testing (1977) showed that it was possible to detect 88 per cent of cases of anencephaly and 79 per cent of cases of open spina bifida if a sample of maternal serum were examined at 16 – 18 weeks of pregnancy. This has now been confirmed by a number of pilot studies (Ferguson-Smith et al., 1978b; Brock et al. 1978; Wald et al., 1979) which use the maternal serum AFP as a voluntary screening test to identify a sample of patients with AFP levels above a given 'cut-off point'. This sample of patients is then investigated further by ultrasonography and amniocentesis, using the amniotic AFP result as the definitive diagnostic test. Causes of false-positive results include multiple pregnancy, missed abortion and overestimated gestation, and most of these can be excluded by ultrasonography. The termination of normal foetuses due to false-positive results is fortunately a rare occurrence (currently less than 1 in 10 000 patients screened). The optimal time for testing has been found to be during the seventeenth week of pregnancy, for the false-negative rate is unacceptably high before 16 completed weeks and after 20 weeks. Thus the screening programme requires close co-ordination and adequate ultrasound facilities for the accurate dating of pregnancies and for safe amniocentesis.

The Department of Health and Social Services and the Scottish Home and Health Department, have each convened working groups to consider the feasibility of mounting national maternal serum AFP screening programmes. It is of interest to note that even before the two working groups had reported, some 48 per cent of all pregnancies in Scotland were tested in 1978 (Table II) and, in England and Wales, routine screening was provided in one or more districts in 46 per cent of all regions (Wald, personal communication). It seems likely that voluntary serum AFP screening will also receive the approval of the Health Department and will soon become part of routine antenatal care in the United Kingdom. As far as is known, this form of screening has not been started to any great extent in other countries in Europe, and is confined to only a few centres in North America.

It has been possible to determine the overall effects of serum AFP screening on the prevalence at birth of neural tube defects in the West of Scotland. Screening started in May, 1975 and in 1978 it was estimated that 56 per cent of the 36 000 births had been screened at between 16 and 20 weeks gestation. Before 1979, our screening policy has been to use a high cut-off point (between the 98th and 99th percentile) to maintain the number of false-positives and thus the number of amniocenteses to manageable proportions, and at the same time reduce the chances of terminating normal pregnancies. We have regarded this as a practical policy until local obstetric services were fully familiar with the requirements of the programme and had experience of amniocentesis. The disadvantage of a high cut-off point is that the sensitivity of the test is reduced and this is reflected in a relatively high false-negative rate. Despite the limitations of this policy, our screening programme in 1978 appears to have reduced the number of anencephalic and spina bifida births in the West of Scotland by 51 per cent and 23 per cent respectively. This reduction has already had a noticeable effect on the local perinatal mortality rate. The 'cut-off' point for 1979 has been dropped to the 97th percentile and this has already produced an improvement in the detection rate for spina bifida, although there has been the expected increase in the number of amniocenteses. However, the obstetric services seem to be responding adequately to this increased load without exposing the patient to undue risk.

Table II

Number and proportion of pregnancies screened for neural tube defects in Scotland in 1978

Health board	Screening centre	Total births	Number screened	Percentage screened	Terminations		Terminations/ 1000 screened
					Anenceph.	Sp. bifida	
Grampian Orkney	Aberdeen[a]	7 695	2 104	27·3	3	1	1·9
Tayside	Dundee[a]	4 700	3 290	70·0	6	8	4·3
Lothians Borders Fife	Edinburgh[a]	14 400	6 138	42·6	7	4	1·8
Ayrshire and Arran Argyll and Clyde Greater Glasgow Lanarkshire Forth Valley Dumfries & Galloway	Glasgow	36 100	20 208	56·0	46	21	3·3
Western Isles Shetland Highland	Not covered	3 050	0	—	—	—	—
Totals		65 945	31 740	48·1	62	34	3·1

[a] Unpublished: Information kindly supplied by Dr H. Thom, Dr J. Crawford and Dr J Scrimgeour, respectively.

Although the proportion of patients who are screened varies markedly among the 14 maternity hospitals which use our screening programme, the overall number continues to increase. Some hospitals achieve over 80 per cent participation, but, once again, the main problem seems to be that many patients do not attend for antenatal care in time to be tested. This group appears to contain a greater proportion of women at higher risk due to their socio-economic condition and higher parity.

The results of the antenatal serum AFP pilot studies have thus been extremely promising. It seems reasonable to predict that if they were applied on a national scale, the birth incidence of open neural tube defects would be reduced by about 75 per cent. It makes sound sense to use them first in areas of high incidence. As with all other forms of family planning, the screening programme should continue to be entirely voluntary for the patient and thus implies that adequate facilities for counselling should be provided. At present, it seems that only a small proportion of the population decline the serum screening test — approximately 5 per cent in the West of Scotland, but apparently less than 1 per cent in South-East Scotland (Brock *et al.*, 1978).

Inborn Errors of Metabolism

Despite the considerable literature which has accumulated on opportunities for prenatal diagnosis of metabolic disease, the effects of such tests can be expected to make comparatively little impact on the total numbers of births affected in the UK. This is because only a small number of pregnancies can be identified from family studies as being at risk of a detectable inborn error. One estimate places the total number of such pregnancies in the UK as between 107 and 120 per annum, of which about one quarter may be expected to be affected (Benson and Polani, quoted in Ferguson-Smith *et al.*, 1978b). Although for each individual family it is important that prenatal diagnosis is available, the numbers involved are clearly not comparable to the numbers at risk each year for chromosome aberrations and neural tube defects. The CGS Survey showed that in 1976, 19 foetuses with inborn errors were detected among 70 pregnancies tested. The widespread interest in this aspect of prenatal diagnosis is indicated by the fact that 12 different laboratories took part in investigating these 70 pregnancies, and also that such a comparatively high proportion of pregnancies recognized as being at risk were tested.

The annual number of pregnancies tested for inborn errors would be increased dramatically if reliable population screening for heterozygotes of the more common autosomal recessive disorders like cystic fibrosis were available. This procedure would aim to identify matings at risk of producing an affected pregnancy so that prenatal diagnosis could be arranged prospectively. Unfortunately, the biochemical defect in cystic fibrosis remains elusive and there are, as yet, no other common single gene defects suitable for this approach, with the single exception of Tay–Sachs disease. Attempts at screening for this disorder among the Ashkenazi Jewish population have been partially successful in North America (Kaback et al., 1974), but have met with a poor response in South East England. Outside the UK, sickle cell disease and the thalassaemias are the most common single gene disorders amenable to heterozygote testing and prenatal diagnosis. Up to comparatively recently, prenatal diagnosis of these conditions depended on foetal blood sampling and analysis of globin chain synthesis (Kan et al., 1975; 1976a; Alter et al., 1976). For a proportion of cases of sickle cell disease and those types of thalassaemia resulting from gene deletion, the techniques of DNA molecular hybridization and restriction enzyme mapping can now be used on DNA preparations derived from samples of amniotic fluid cells (Kan et al., 1976b; Kan and Dozy, 1978). Development of these techniques holds great hope for the prenatal diagnosis of other single gene defects in the future. In the meantime, only a comparatively small number of thalassaemic families receive the benefit of prenatal diagnosis, and the major requirement at present is to train adequate numbers of staff to provide the service that is urgently needed, particularly in countries bordering the Mediterranean and in South East Asia where the problem is immense.

Miscellaneous Disorders

Most other disorders for which prenatal diagnosis is currently available are not sufficiently common to make much impact on the birth incidence of congenital malformations and genetic disease. Among them are the developmental disorders recognizable by ultrasonic examination and foetoscopy. Both procedures are in a rapid phase of technological development and we must expect many additions in the near future to the gross disorders at present detectable.

The development of ultrasonography for this work is particularly encouraging as it is a non-invasive procedure without apparent harm to either mother or foetus. My hope is that it may soon replace amniocentesis and amniotic AFP investigation as the diagnostic test in the spina bifida screening programmes, so that we can avoid the foetal loss which complicates a small proportion of amniocentesis cases. At present, in skilled hands, over 75 per cent of open neural tube defects can be diagnosed by sonar scanning, as can such other foetal malformations as polycystic kidney, renal agenesis, exomphalos, short-limbed dwarfism and microcephaly. However, the procedure is time-consuming and there are too few experienced operators to provide a routine screening service.

The foetal loss rate following foetoscopy is much higher than following amniocentesis, the more experienced centres quoting a rate of about 7 per cent (Fairweather, 1978). Foetoscopy is thus only indicated where the pregnancy is at high risk of serious foetal abnormality as, for example, in thalassaemia where the recurrence risk is 25 per cent. Although direct visualization of foetal abnormality is possible, current needlescopes have too small a range of vision to make external examination of the foetus easy. Its main value lies in its use in obtaining blood samples for such procedures as globin chain examination in the haemoglobinopathies, Factor VIII assay in haemophilia (Mibashan et al., 1979), and CPK estimation in Duchenne muscular dystrophy (the reliability of the latter is uncertain and more research is required before its application). Once the safety of foetoscopy has been improved, the prospect of using foetal blood samples for the prenatal diagnosis of a number of additional haematological and biochemical disorders will be realized. It may even become possible to test for a number of single gene defects through genetic linkage with common blood group or red cell enzyme markers, but this will depend on expansion of the human gene map, for only a few disorders are amenable to this strategy at present. These include a small proportion of cases of myotonic dystrophy (linked to the secretor locus), a few haemophilia families (in which suitable variants of the X-linked glucose-6-phosphate dehydrogenase locus are segregating) and cases of the 21-hydroxylase deficient form of congenital adrenal hyperplasia (closely linked to the major histocompatibility locus on chromosome 6).

The Reliability and Safety of Prenatal Diagnosis

This brief review of the applications of prenatal diagnosis, its present effect and future potential for the reduction of certain birth defects, would be incomplete without some mention of the problems that have to be faced before the procedure is fully acceptable to the public. A major requirement is that it must be seen to be both reliable and safe and it is clear that any nationally approved service must have adequate quality control and the means to monitor the outcome of its work. The results of the MRC Report on the Hazards of Amniocentesis (1978) suggest that the foetal loss attributable to amniocentesis is about $1-1.5$ per cent of those tested, with an additional infant morbidity (mainly respiratory and orthopaedic problems) in $1-1.5$ per cent. This study is based on data from a number of centres with differing experience and expertise, and once amniocentesis has been confined solely to centres of excellence it is expected that these figures can be improved. However, it is essential that each centre continues to have a local monitoring scheme. The CGS Study found that in 1976 only a minority of prenatal diagnostic laboratories were able to follow up their results adequately, and most had no measure of the reliability and safety of their work. Adequate monitoring is time-consuming and administrators responsible for health service resources appear unsympathetic to requests for staffing and financial support for such work. In the West of Scotland, all amniocentesis cases are followed to delivery and a routine search is made among labour room, nursery and surgical paediatric records for false-negative results in our maternal serum AFP screening programme. This task is becoming increasingly laborious as the numbers of patients increase. Efforts are therefore being made to computerize our laboratory results so that they can be linked centrally with maternity in-patient records. The success of this scheme will depend on how far it is possible to record accurate details of each birth on the forms used to collect maternity in-patient statistics. If central monitoring is found to be impractical, far better facilities than are at present available (including adequate staffing) will have to be provided for local monitoring.

Summary

Prenatal diagnosis is acceptable to all but a small proportion of the community and sufficient evidence has accumulated over the past ten years to show that it can appreciably reduce the birth incidence of certain severe congenital malformations and genetic defects. The most dramatic effect on birth incidence is seen for open neural tube defects in regions where maternal serum AFP screening is employed. For example, in the West of Scotland, the overall reduction in all major malformations of the central nervous system achieved by screening 56 per cent of the pregnant population in 1978 was in the order of 37 per cent, and this proportion is increasing. Where the indication for prenatal diagnosis is the risk of chromosome aberration due to advancing maternal age, progress has been slower. In 1976 the birth incidence of Down's syndrome in the UK appears to have been reduced by this means by only 3 per cent. If all women 35 years of age and over had undergone amniocentesis the expected reduction would have been 37 per cent: however, only about 6 per cent of women in this age group were tested. It appears that the lack of facilities is holding up the development of a service which will adequately fulfil the needs of the community. In addition, a more strenuous approach is required towards reducing the proportion of women attending for antenatal care too late to be given the option of prenatal diagnosis.

There are at present too few pregnancies identifiable as being at risk of single gene defects in the UK to expect prenatal diagnosis to lead to a major reduction in affected births. In countries where thalassaemia and the haemoglobinopathies are common, prenatal diagnostic services are not yet developed sufficiently to make any impact, although the potential for the future is enormous.

References

Alberman, E., Berry, A.C. and Polani, P.E. (1979). Planning an amniocentesis service for Down syndrome. *Lancet*, i 50.

Alter, B.P., Modell, C.B., Fairweather, D., Hobbins, J.G. *et al.* (1976). Prenatal diagnosis of haemoglobinopathies. A review of 15 cases. *New England Journal of Medicine*, 295, 1437–1443.

Brock, D.J.H. and Sutcliffe, R.G. (1972). Alpha-fetoprotein in the antenatal diagnosis of anencephaly and spina bifida. *Lancet*, ii, 197–199.

Brock, D.J.H., Scrimgeour, J.B., Steven, J., Baron, L. and Watt, M. (1978). Maternal plasma alpha-fetoprotein screening for fetal neural tube defects. *British Journal of Obstetrics and Gynaecology*, 85, 575–581.

Carter, C.O. and Evans, K.A. (1979). Amniocentesis and the alpha-fetoprotein screening programme. *Lancet*, i, 40.

Evans, J., Hunter, A.G.W. and Hamerton, J.L. (1978). Down's syndrome and recent demographic trends in Manitoba. *Journal of Medical Genetics*, 15, 43–47.

Fairweather, D.V.I. (1978). Television medicine. *British Medical Journal*, i, 503–504.

Ferguson-Smith, M.A. (1965). Chromosome aberrations in developmental disease and their familial transmission. In *Biological Aspects of Social Problems*, edited by J.E. Meade and A.S. Parkes, pp. 152–163. Edinburgh: Oliver & Boyd.

Ferguson-Smith, M.A. (1979). Maternal age specific incidence of chromosome aberrations at amniocentesis. In *Proceedings of the Third European Conference on Prenatal Diagnosis of Genetic Disorders*, edited by J.D. Murken, S. Stengel-Rutkowski, and E. Schwinger, pp. 1–14. Stuttgart: Enke.

Ferguson-Smith, M.A., Benson, P.F., Brock, D.J.H., Fairweather, D.V.I., Harris, R., Laurence, K.H., McDermott, A., Patrick, A.D., Polani, P.E. and Walker, S. (1978a). The provision of services for the prenatal diagnosis of fetal abnormality in the United Kingdom. *Bulletin of the Eugenics Society*, Supplement 3, 1–33.

Ferguson-Smith, M.A., Rawlinson, H.A., May, H.M., Tait, H.A., Vince, J.D., Gibson, A.A.M., Robinson, H.P., and Ratcliffe, J.G. (1978b). Avoidance of anencephalic and spina bifida births by maternal serum alpha-fetoprotein screening. *Lancet* i,1330–1333.

Hagard, S. and Carter, F.A. (1976). The prevention of Down's syndrome births: a cost-benefit analysis. *British Medical Journal*, i, 753–756.

Kaback, M.M., Zeiger, R.S., Reynolds, L.W. and Sonneborn, M. (1974). Tay–Sachs disease: a model for the control of recessive genetic disorders. In *Proceedings of the Fourth International Conference on Birth Defects*, edited by A.G. Motulsky and W. Lenz., pp. 248–262. Amsterdam: Exerpta Medica.

Kan, Y.W. and Dozy, A.M. (1978). Polymorphism of DNA sequence adjacent to human ß globin structural gene: Relationship to sickle mutation. *Proceedings of the National Academy of Sciences*, 75, 5631–35.

Kan, Y.W., Golbus, M.S., Klein, P. and Dozy, A.M. (1975). Successful application of prenatal diagnosis in a pregnancy at risk for homozygous ß Thalassaemia. *New England Journal of Medicine*, 292, 1096.

Kan, Y.W., Golbus, M.S., and Dozy, A.M. (1976a). Prenatal diagnosis of ß Thalassaemia. Clinical application of molecular hybridisation. *New England Journal of Medicine*, 295, 1165–1167.

Kan, Y.W., Golbus, M.S. and Trecartin, R. (1976b). Prenatal diagnosis of sickle cell anaemia. *New England Journal of Medicine*, 294, No. 19, 1039.

Mibashan, R.S., Rodeck, C.H., Thumpston, J.K., Edwards R.J., Singer, J.D., White, J.M. and Campbell, S. (1979). Plasma assay of fetal factors VIIIC and IX for prenatal diagnosis of haemophilia. *Lancet*, i, 1309–1311.

MRC Working Party on Amniocentesis (1978). An assessment of the hazards of amniocentesis. *British Journal of Obstetrics and Gynaecology*, 85, Supplement 2, 1–41.

Murken, J.D., Stengel-Rutkowski, S. and Schwinger, E. (1979). Prenatal diagnosis of genetic disorders. *Proceedings of the Third European Conference on Prenatal Diagnosis*, Stuttgart: Enke.

Riis, P. and Fuchs, F. (1960). Antenatal determination of fetal sex in prevention of hereditary diseases. *Lancet*, ii, 180.

Steele, M.W. and Breg, W.R. (1966). Chromosome analysis of human amniotic fluid cells. *Lancet*, i, 383–385.

U.K. Collaborative Study (1977). Maternal serum alphafetoprotein measurement in antenatal screening for anencephaly and spina bifida in early pregnancy. *Lancet*, i, 1323–1332.

Wald, N.J., Cuckle, H.S., Boreham, J., Brett, R., Stirrat, G.M., Bennett, M.J., Turnbull, A.L., Solymar, M., Jones, N., Bobrow, M. and Evans, C.J. (1979). Antenatal screening in Oxford for fetal neural tube defects. *British Journal of Obstetrics and Gynaecology*, 86, 91–100.

Effects of Drugs in Pregnancy and During Lactation

D.F. HAWKINS

Institute of Obstetrics and Gynaecology, Hammersmith Hospital, London, England

The thalidomide disaster of twenty years ago had a number of beneficial sequelae. The publicity that occurred, and still occurs whenever the media focus on one of the people who were born with a thalidomide deformity, leads patients to question the need for and safety of any drugs they are asked to take in pregnancy. Doctors have become more circumspect in their prescribing for pregnant patients and most have strong reservations about the use of new drugs in pregnancy. In addition there has been a tremendous expansion in laboratory research on animals dealing with the demonstration of drug-induced teratogenic phenomena and their mechanisms.

Inevitably, the emotional context has led to over-reaction, and this in turn has led to exploitation. Policies of therapeutic nihilism are common and refusal to prescribe or accept harmless asymptomatic medicines during pregnancy leads to unnecessary suffering by patients, and withholding of specific remedies sometimes gives rise to serious consequences. The medico-legal implications have been taken to heart by the pharmaceutical houses and very large sums of money are spent on laboratory and animal tests for teratogenesis which are largely irrelevant to potential risks in human pregnancy. This is partly necessitated by the requirements of the Committee on Safety of Medicines for acceptance of a new drug which may be used in pregnancy. The more background information available about a new drug the better, but the exercise is really undertaken so that justice is seen to be done. It ignores the fact that a potential human teratogen can slip through the screening net, whilst many drugs that might be harmless and of value in human therapeutics are shelved. The cost of the investigations is very considerable and severely limits the introduction of new therapeutic agents. This might not be a bad thing but the prices of the drugs that are introduced are also inflated. Another form of protective over-reaction by the pharmaceutical companies lies in the provision of warnings and contraindications in data sheets (Association of the British Pharmaceutical Industry, 1980) which are sometimes out of proportion to any known risk and sometimes contraindicate the administration of an agent of known safety. One can hardly blame the drug industry for taking such precautions. The sums of money for which they can be sued are enormous and decisions are based on legal principles rather than everyday commonsense attribution of fault. Should the fullest implications of 'strict liability' become embodied in the law, then he who made the drug may become responsible for not only the damage wreaked by its misuse but also the consequences of predictable side-effects in a small proportion of patients (British Medical Journal, 1979). The financial consequences of such a situation could cripple the pharmaceutical industry and prevent development of important new drugs.

The Congenital Disabilities (Civil Liability) Act, 1976, passed into law unnoticed by the majority of medical practitioners. Under this Act, a child born with a disability can sue the mother's doctor for any action which caused the disability. With the logic of expediency, if the congenital abnormality is such that the child is stillborn, there is no recourse under the Act. The medical practitioner is protected against a civil action if he took reasonable care in relation to established medical practice at the time he gave a drug, he should inform the parents of any risk to the foetus. It is possible that a doctor who deliberately did not convey such information about a small risk, because of the anxiety it might cause, would find the fact that he acted in good faith in the interests of his patient an adequate defence.

Another aspect of exploitation of the teratogenic potential of drugs occurs with women who desire a therapeutic abortion. In fact there are very few therapeutic agents which are major teratogens and could reasonably be held to cause a "substantial risk that if the child were born it would . . . be seriously handicapped" under the terms of the Abortion Act, 1967. For example, the risk to the foetus of a woman who has taken chloroquine for malaria is probably 1 in 100 or less and of a woman who has had an oral hormonal pregnancy test (Greenberg et al., 1977) 1 in 1000 or less, and these can not be regarded as substantial risks in the context of the Act. When the very small degree of risk has been explained to the patient and she continues to exploit it, there is usually another reason why she wants her pregnancy terminated. Though this may be apparent to the doctor, it may sometimes not even be recognized by the patient herself. Pregnancies are sometimes terminated in consequence, the patient remaining unaware that the legal grounds are her anxiety rather than risk of teratogenesis. This can have medico-legal consequences. In a recent case (Medical Defence Union, 1979) a woman was scheduled for an X-ray hysterocervicogram, presumably because she desired a pregnancy. Doubts about her last menstrual period were not resolved and it subsequently transpired that she was probably pregnant when she had the X-ray examination. The exposure to the foetus must have been of the order of 2 to 5 rads; a minimum exposure of 50 rads is the level at which there could be considered a probable relationship between irradiation and foetal damage (Sternberg, 1973). None the less, 'because of the irradiation risk to the foetus' the pregnancy was terminated. The fact that the indication for the abortion was invalid passed unnoticed, and the patient was awarded £1824 damages and costs on the basis that the performance of the X-rays led to the need for termination of the pregnancy! It is therefore vital that when a pregnancy is terminated in circumstances like this that it be made abundantly clear to the patient that the grounds are her anxiety, and that real risk to the foetus is not 'substantial'.

It is clearly of great importance that wherever possible the magnitude of the real risk associated with a potentially teratogenic exposure be available to doctors and laymen alike. In practice this risk is seldom known and with the great majority of drugs that have been suspected hard evidence of a causal relationship is lacking.

Difficulties in the Assessment of Teratogenesis in Humans

Test conditions in experimental programmes aimed at recognizing teratogens differ fundamentally from those pertaining in human therapeutics. Short-term exposures of chick embryos or pregnant rodents to large doses of drugs must be expected to produce results which differ from those encountered in clinical practice. There is also the problem of species difference. For example, the rat foetus is immune to the teratogenic effects of thalidomide or cortisone which are demonstrable under experimental conditions, whilst mouse and rabbit foetuses are highly susceptible (Tuchmann-Duplessis, 1965). As a result screening procedures can at most suggest either that a given compound or group of compounds have a tendency to be teratogenic in some species greater than that of other drugs, or, rarely, that there is a specific influence on a given organ system or metabolic process. The last finding is of the most interest; if a mode of action is known then detailed experimental assessment of possible relevance to humans becomes feasible. The most worrying possibility with respect to a new drug is that it might be innocuous in screening tests and yet be teratogenic in humans.

A great deal of the suggestions that some drugs might be causing increases in congenital abnormality rates arise from retrospective studies based on large numbers of patients. A major difficulty in work of this sort is the biased recall of patients. A woman who has had an abnormal baby will remember every aspirin she took during the pregnancy and sometimes apparently recall taking medication that she did not actually have. In contrast, the woman who has had a normal pregnancy forgets a lot of the medicines she has ingested. The same phenomenon applies to the doctors prescribing the drugs. Reference to case notes does not eliminate this problem — abnormal pregnancies are more fully documented and antenatal care divided between hospitals and family practitioners ensures that records are incomplete. There is a real need for well-planned prospective studies in which great pains are taken to avoid bias in selection of patients. Really adequate prospective studies are expensive in time, personnel and money to run properly and they take years to produce results. Even then, they are not secure from the effects of failure of patient compliance in taking drugs as prescribed, or from the effects of self-medication.

A weakness of epidemiological studies is that they commonly depend on correlation analysis. Because two attributes are correlated, it does not necessarily mean that they are causally related. It has been pointed out in relation to cigarette smoking in pregnancy that the association between addiction to haggis and a liking for the music of the bagpipes does not mean that indulgence in the former delicacy causes a predilection for cacophony (Hawkins, 1959). In order to give any strength to the argument, a causal mechanism must be demonstrated. Whilst it is well established that cigarette smoking in pregnancy is associated with small increases in the incidences of intra-uterine growth retardation, premature labour and perinatal mortality, it is only now, 20 years later, that there is good evidence of possible mechanisms — reduced oxygen availability (Davies et al., 1979) and placental damage (Naeye, 1978). Even then, it is possible that there is substance in Yerushalmy's (1971) contention that smokers differ in their environmental, behavioural and biological characteristics, and the observed differences are due to the smoker, not the smoking. Although Butler et al. (1972) found that women who gave up smoking by the fourth month of pregnancy had an improved prognosis, Donovan (1977), in a randomized controlled trial showed that women who are persuaded to give up smoking in pregnancy obtain no such improvement. It may be (Hawkins, 1976), that we are dealing with two different types of women, the former group being distinguished by their exhibiting a pica. In another context the demonstration by Janerich and others (1974) of a very small risk of limb-reduction defects in the babies of women who become pregnant whilst taking oral contraceptives was given the ring of truth by the fact that all six of the affected babies were male, suggesting a specific mode of action.

Another requirement for establishing the validity of an apparent association is that the nature of the abnormality be consistent with the stage of gestation at which the presumed teratogenic insult was applied. For example, at about 35 days from the last menstrual period, thalidomide can cause ear defects; the major limb dysplasias occur when it is given at about 50 days (Lenz, 1965). Phocomelia cannot be attributed to thalidomide given late in pregnancy, after the limbs are fully formed. In general, susceptibility to any teratogenic stimulus tends to be related to the organ system developing at the time the stimulus is applied. A slightly increased incidence of congenital malformations was found by Nelson and Forfar (1971) in mothers taking barbiturates in the first trimester of pregnancy. The Royal College of General Practitioners (1975) found a similar association, mainly with minor defects, but when they tried to correlate the findings with respect to the nature of the defect and the duration of gestation at which the drugs were given, there was no suggestion of a cause and effect relationship.

The next problem is that of interaction with other agents. The retrospective study of Stewart et al. (1958) concluded that a child whose mother had had an abdominal X-ray during pregnancy was twice as likely to die of malignant disease before the age of ten as a child not so exposed. Other authors subsequently cast doubt on the findings (Court Brown et al., 1960; Magnin, 1962). None the less, the work had such an effect that over the next few years it was estimated that three times as many babies as had been stated to be at risk were lost because necessary X-rays were withheld. It may be recalled that Fedrick and Alberman (1972) showed that maternal influenza in pregnancy is associated with an incidence of 4 per 1000 of leukaemia and related conditions in the offspring, and that confirmatory observations have since been published (Bithell et al., 1973; Hakulinen et al., 1973). Should this association be causal, it could account for a high proportion of the total incidence of leukaemia in childhood. When it is considered that many of these women had X-rays in pregnancy, and the possibility that sub-clinical virus infections might also be involved, the difficulty in drawing any valid conclusion about an X-ray effect is extreme. Where there has been any sort of epidemic situation, subsequent studies of congenital abnormalities are confounded by the question of a possible association possibly being due to the drug or to the disease it was given to cure. On a more general level, these may be the explanation of the apparent discrepancy between Nelson and Forfar's (1971) finding with barbiturates and the Royal College of General Practitioners' (1975) demonstration that the drugs did not seem to be acting as teratogens. Even Smithells' (1976) definitive review of the information on anti-epileptic drugs does not completely overcome this problem. He showed that epileptics taking the drugs had a congenital abnormality rate of 6 per cent, compared with 1 − 4 per cent in epileptics not on treatment. It must still be conceded that the epileptics taking the drugs would be the more severe cases, and the disease itself might be the causative agent.

Genetic and environmental factors may be the basis of real or apparent associations with implications of teratogenicity. Apart from the factor of species difference, it may be that some populations are unduly susceptible to such effects. There is no clear evidence that this is the case in humans, but the high incidence of anencephaly and central nervous system defects in the north-west of England (with a high proportion of women of Irish origin), South Wales and Southern Ireland suggests that people of Celtic origin may have a genetic susceptibility to malformations of the nervous system. The first convincing study linking synthetic sex steroids with a very small risk of congenital abnormality came from New York State, where the link was with limb reduction defects (Janerich et al., 1974). Nora and Nora's (1975) work on the same theme, from Colorado, emphasized a syndrome of multiple congenital abnormalities, involving vertebral, anal, cardiac, tracheo-oesophageal and renal anomalies, as well as limb defects. Other environmental situations seem to have ill-defined effects which create great difficulty in analysis. Studies based on mailed questionnaires, with their positive bias, have suggested that pregnant lady anaesthetists have an increased abortion and congenital abnormality rate (Corbett et al., 1974; Tomlin, 1979). Though there are statistical defects in these studies (Vessey, 1979), it is known that large doses of some anaesthetic agents are teratogenic in animals under laboratory conditions (Smith, 1974) and there is even a suggestion that women exposed to organic solvents in industry have an increased congenital abnormality rate (Holmberg, 1979). The problem in interpretation lies in the fact that abortion and congenital abnormality rates are equally high in the wives of male anaesthetists (Tomlin, 1979) and that lady anaesthetists who do not work in pregnancy and lady doctors in general also have high spontaneous abortion and congenital abnormality rates (Knill-Jones et al., 1972). The fact that Tomlin's (1979) data were derived solely from the West Midlands has already been introduced into the argument (McPherson et al., 1978), and we await with confidence the suggestion that fluoridation of tap water has something to do with it! Whilst it is highly desirable that atmospheric pollution of operating theatres by anaesthetic gases should be reduced, the evidence that these agents are a hazard to pregnant personnel is tenuous (Smith, 1974) and, in the current state of knowledge, any ill-effects recorded may be due to factors inherent in the population at risk (Hawkins and Love, 1978).

A final problem with which the seeker after truth has to contend in the jungle of inadequate information about human teratogenesis is the attitude of those who contribute to the literature. Ever since the thalidomide tragedy there seems to have been a premium on being the first to suggest or report a possibility of teratogenesis. Every sympathy must be given to the desire not to fail to make an association known. At the same time, ill-founded reports cause extensive confusion in the literature and their interpretation defies the average doctor. The medico-legal potential of the reports is very considerable and the amounts of money which might be involved are massive. Finally, it often takes many years of intensive and expensive study to refute even a vague and tenuous assertion. Looking dispassionately at the drugs which have been challenged in this way, one cannot help but wonder if subtle and far-reaching commercial influences are at work, even though those who make the reports are above suspicion. The target drugs are usually very widely used agents which have been available for many years and upon which profits are often small. It is strange how often a more recently developed alternative with commercial rather than real medical advantages seems to be available!

An example of the 'theoretical possibility' is the suggestion which appeared five years ago that sulphonamides are contraindicated in pregnancy because they interfere with the foetal enzymes which conjugate bilirubin and cause kernicterus in the newborn. It seems a surprising contention, in view of the fact that literally millions of pregnant women have been treated with sulphonamides over the last 40 years without apparent harm to their babies. Investigation reveals a complete lack of valid reports in the literature associating maternal soluble sulphonamide therapy with neonatal kernicterus, and no cases have been reported to the Committee on Safety of Medicines in 20 years. The answer is that in clinical practice the problem of newborn sulphonamide intoxication does not arise. Soluble sulphonamides are rapidly excreted in pregnancy, and they are not used in labour because they are then not absorbed by the oral route and they are painful if given intramuscularly. Nonetheless, the statement that sulphonamides are contraindicated in pregnancy has crept into some authoritative articles and even textbooks.

A more recent and extraordinary suggestion concerned the use of metronidazole in pregnancy, a drug which was exonerated after suggestions had been made that it might be teratogenic (see Hawkins, 1976; Morgan, 1978), following its introduction in an oral form to a competitive market in the United States of America. Large doses of metronidazole, of the order of 2g/day, can interact with alcohol metabolism causing the accumulation of acetaldehyde, which has toxic effects — an action similar to that of disulfiram, only metronidazole is not nearly so effective or consistent as disulfiram. One of the theories of the mechanism of the foetal alcohol syndrome — which is extremely rare in Great Britain — is that it is a toxic effect of the catabolite acetaldehyde. It was recently suggested that the use of metronidazole in pregnancy is contraindicated, because if it caused accumulation of acetaldehyde, and if this was the mechanism of the foetal alcohol syndrome, and if the patient were an undetected alcoholic, then it might increase the chance of an alcohol syndrome baby! What tortuous thinking! The incidence of alcoholism in pregnancy in my clinic, in a poor area of West London where we have had a special interest in detecting this condition, is less than 1 in 500; multiply by the incidence of trichomoniasis, of the order of 5 per cent, and we only have 1 in 10 000, or 1 patient at risk every 20 years, even if the hypothesis were true. In fact we have not delivered a foetal alcohol baby at Hammersmith or Queen Charlotte's Maternity Hospital in ten years, encompassing some 50 000 deliveries. The effort given to indicting metronidazole would have been better devoted to detecting alcoholism in pregnancy and giving the patients B vitamins and protein supplements, or to advising patients not to drink excess alcohol whilst taking metronidazole.

In addition to attempting to evaluate isolated case reports of coincidental associations between administration of drugs and an abnormal foetus, we have to cope with the 'me too' syndrome mentioned by Smithells (1976). A year or two ago it was suggested that foetal abnormality could result from a pregnancy which occurred in the presence of a copper intra-uterine contraceptive device. In one of the two cases presented, it seemed likely that the device had been expelled before the pregnancy occurred. The device was a Graffenberg ring which only contains small amounts of copper and could probably only release amounts less than those normally present in uterine fluid. Inevitably, within a few weeks there were reports of two further similar coincidences in the correspondence columns of the journal concerned. Fortunately, records were available of sufficient cases of pregnancy occurring in copper device patients (Snowden, 1976) to dispel the idea that the association was real.

Most recently, we have to deal with an *ex cathedra* recommendation from the Committee on the Review of Medicines (1979) that the use of barbiturates is contraindicated in pregnancy. Barbiturates are drugs which have been widely used in pregnancy for 50 years without significant harm, apart from the occasional maternal skin rash. Fifteen years ago I recall being warned that they might interfere with the baby's liver function. Ten years ago we were advised that this was a good thing, in that the adaptive enzymes thereby stimulated tended to prevent newborn hyperbilirubinaemia and even neonatal asphyxia. More recently, it was said that it would warp the baby's psyche if barbiturates were taken by the mother during pregnancy. It is not surprising that the last suggestion was greeted by obstetricians with a complete lack of reaction. We know that barbiturates used in large doses throughout pregnancy to treat epilepsy may carry the same small risk of teratogenesis as other anti-epileptic drugs (Speidel and Meadow, 1972), and that this risk might be reduced by giving folic acid supplements. We know that large doses of barbiturates taken by epileptics or addicts shortly before labour can lead to a withdrawal syndrome which requires careful management of the newborn, as is the case with other anticonvulsants, including opiates and benzodiazepines (British Medical Journal, 1972). We know that in general use in sedative doses, barbiturates, in common with benzodiazepines, have been accused of teratogenesis and subsequently exonerated. We know that we do not generate barbiturate addicts by short term use in pregnancy for a defined purpose. How then, are we to cope reasonably with such a recommendation by the Committee on the Review of Medicines, with its authority and medico-legal implications, its failure to present any evidence, and its suggestion that we should use benzodiazepines instead?

The Clinical Decision

Faced with all these problems, the clinician frequently confronts the need for making a decision on the use of drugs in pregnancy. Somehow he must come to a conclusion which conveys the smallest possible risk to foetal development but does not withhold essential treatment from the mother and does not place the foetus at risk by failure to treat a maternal or obstetric disorder. He may arrive at a satisfactory answer by considering some basic rules of prescribing in pregnancy, by generating a sense of perspective as to which information should be applied to policy-making and which to the management of the individual patient, and finally by considering drugs in pregnancy in three categories: major teratogens, therapeutic agents whose use may incur a small teratogenic risk, and drugs at which the finger of suspicion has been pointed but which have not been demonstrated to be harmful.

PRESCRIBING IN PREGNANCY

Whenever a drug is given to a pregnant or a possibly pregnant woman, the prescription should be assessed as to whether or not treatment is really necessary. A second consideration should be as to whether or not alternative therapy, not using drugs, might be efficacious. The pre-packed tablet is all too readily available and the virtues of dietetic management and of physical medicine, psychotherapy and simple rest too easily forgotten.

It is preferable when prescribing in pregnancy to use drugs which have been widely used in pregnancy for many years, rather than recently introduced agents with ill-established or merely theoretical advantages.

Whenever a drug is used which is known or even suspected to be associated with some teratogenic risk, careful thought should be given to measures which might attenuate that risk. In general, if it is reasonable to postpone treatment until the second trimester, as in the case of a mild anaemia or an asymptomatic trichomonal infection, then this should be done.

The index of suspicion should be high with every female between the ages of fourteen and forty-eight, when a drug is prescribed — might she be pregnant? With patients suffering from medical disorders considera-tion of the patient's reproductive plans and the likelihood of unplanned reproduction should be assessed at the start of treatment. She must be told that if there is any chance of pregnancy then her treatment should be reviewed before she ever conceives. The discussion can be renewed in relation to contraceptive precautions each time she is seen. The physician then has a chance to have the hypertensive woman on drugs which are easiest to handle in pregnancy, to get the thyrotoxic to have her partial thyroidectomy performed and be on the minimum of drugs, and to have the psychiatric patient on agents known to be harmless, before they ever conceive. He is able to have the epileptic on the lowest reasonable dose of drugs together with folic acid supplements when she conceives and the chronic bronchitic on ampicillin instead of a tetra-cycline in early pregnancy.

POLICY AND THE INDIVIDUAL PATIENT

Having learned to take all possible precautions the physician must then develop a sense of perspective in interpreting the warnings to which he is frequently exposed, both in the medical literature and by the media. Such pronouncements are fairly readily classified as to whether they concern general policies or a real risk to the individual patient.

The classification can first be made according to the magnitude of the risk. One is then in a position to decide never to use synthetic sex hormones as an oral pregnancy test as a matter of policy, and at the same time to reassure the woman who has been given such a test that the odds are at the very least 500 to 1 that the foetus will be unaffected. Similarly, one can advise the pregnant patient that in general smoking and over-indulgence in alcohol are bad for her health and that of the baby, as a matter of policy. At the same time it is possible to reassure the woman who finds it difficult to reduce her smoking below 10 cigarettes a day that the risk to the baby is very small (Butler *et al.*, 1972) and probably preventable by good obstetric care, that the chance of doing any good by abstinence enforced in pregnancy is debatable (Donovan, 1977), and that the alternatives of tranquillizers and sedatives may be equally harmful. The patient whose alcohol consumption does not exceed six measures of spirits a day may be told that she is not even in the usual risk group for intra-uterine growth retardation, let alone for a malformed foetal alcohol baby (Ouellette *et al.*, 1977).

The classification must also take into account the severity of the condition from which the foetus might be at risk. For example, whilst sedatives and hypnotics are best avoided in pregnancy, the small risk of minor lesions which was suggested and then disproved in relation to barbiturates (Royal College of General Practitioners, 1975) should give doctors confidence in dispelling patient anxieties generated by the Committee on the Regulation of Medicines! The hazard of 19-nor-steroids in early pregnancy dignified by the term 'masculinization of the female foetus' was in general a minor degree of hypertrophy of the clitoris which resolved spontaneously in the first year or two of life (Wilkins, 1960) and only very rarely did fusion of the labio-scrotal folds require a snip with a pair of scissors. The policy in the case of habitual abortion in whom progesterone deficiency is demonstrable may be to use a 17-alpha-hydroxy progestagen (Hawkins, 1974), but the woman who has been given a 19-nor-steroid in early pregnancy can be reassured.

One would like to add that the stature of the sources of the information should be of help. Regrettably this is not so; the most learned individuals and eminent organizations have at one time or another fallen into the trap of confusing what should have been a matter of policy with a real risk to the individual.

CLASSES OF TERATOGEN

Classification of human teratogens into three groups is of assistance in making clinical decisions.

The first class may be termed 'major teratogens' and consists of agents which are well-established either to cause a high incidence of foetal abnormalities, or are known to cause some abnormalities and to be non-essential or completely replaceable by a harmless agent during pregnancy. Some examples are shown in Table I.

Table I
Major teratogens in humans

Actinomycin
Alkylating agents
Antimetabolites
Radiochemicals
Tetracycline
Thalidomide
Pelvic irradiation for cancer
Prolonged foetal anoxia; open-heart surgery

Source: modified from Hawkins, 1976.

The second class consists of therapeutic agents which are essential in the management of disorders in pregnancy, but are known to convey a small teratogenic risk. Some of these drugs are indicated in Table II.

The third class are agents which have been accused of teratogenicity without clear evidence and which are in fact widely used without apparent risk.

Major Teratogens in Humans

These agents (Table I) should only be used in the pregnant woman in very exceptional circumstances, the serious risk to the foetus being clearly understood by the patient. With the exception of tetracycline, their use would seem to justify legal abortion in Great Britain, should the foetus survive and abortion be requested by the patient.

ANTIMITOTIC DRUGS

The antimetabolites such as methotrexate, mercaptopurine and fluorouracil, and also actinomycin, convey the greatest risk and it is possible that cytarabine falls in this class. None the less, successful pregnancies have been reported in patients taking mercaptopurine (Merskey and Rigal, 1956; Ravenna and Stein, 1963). With patients to whom

Table II

Some therapeutic agents believed to convey a teratogenic risk in small proportion of cases

Antithyroid drugs; iodides	Foetal goitre
Azathioprine	Susceptibility to virus infection
Barbiturates (large doses)	Newborn withdrawal syndrome
Chloroquine	Retinal damage; rarely, multiple abnormalities
Coumarin anticoagulants	Foetal haemorrhage; rarely, foetal abnormalities
Diazepam and related benzodiazepines (large doses)	Newborn withdrawal syndrome
Frusemide	Maternal intravascular dehydration and reduced placental perfusion leading to foetal growth retardation
Ganglion blockers	Paralytic ileus
Glucocorticoids	Susceptibility to virus infection
Live vaccines	Foetal virus infection
Narcotics	Respiratory depression; newborn withdrawal syndrome
19-Nor-steroids	Virilisation of female foetus (transient clitoral hypertrophy; rarely labial fusion)
Phenytoin, primidone	Foetal abnormalities, foetal bleeding; newborn withdrawal syndrome
Rauwolfia alkaloids	Newborn depression syndrome
Streptomycin, kanamycin, gentamicin, vancomycin, tobramycin	Sometimes minor 8th nerve damage detected on audiometry, very rarely deafness
Vitamin D (large doses); dihydrotachysterol	Skeletal abnormalities

Source: modified from Hawkins, 1976.

therapeutic abortion is not acceptable, it is possible that a regimen including administration of folic acid might convey some protection but it might also interfere with cytoxic efficacy.

The risk to the foetus with alkylating agents such as chlorambucil or busulphan is considerably lower, only some 10 per cent of surviving foetuses being seriously affected.

RADIOCHEMICALS

Radioactive iodine (^{131}I) should not be employed for diagnosis or treatment in pregnancy as there is a serious risk of foetal goitre and there are benign alternatives for most purposes. Radioactive phosphorus also conveys a hazard to foetal bone marrow if the pregnancy continues.

Bone scanning with ^{47}Ca or ^{85}Sr should be forbidden during pregnancy because of the free transfer to the foetus and the avidity of foetal bone for these ions.

TETRACYCLINE

This drug discolours the foetal teeth and causes enamel hypoplasia in the deciduous teeth. Alternative antibiotics are always available. Tetracycline damage to teeth can be distinguished because the teeth fluoresce under ultra-violet illumination.

THALIDOMIDE

Although the maximum susceptibility for major deformities is between 35 and 50 days from the last menstrual period, foetal neurological abnormalities can occur later in pregnancy. The drug should never be used as a sedative in pregnancy.

RADIOTHERAPY

Exposure to 50 rads or more bears a 'probable relationship' to foetal abnormality or abortion (Sternberg, 1973). Abdominal irradiation with 350−400 rads used to be used to induce therapeutic abortion. Pelvic radiation for malignant disease almost always results in abortion or foetal death, but foetuses surviving small doses may be abnormal.

FOETAL ANOXIA

The anoxia in the peripheral circulation associated with open heart surgery and a by-pass circulation has a similar outcome; it is usually requested that therapeutic abortion be performed before the operation.

Therapeutic Agents Used in Pregnancy Which May Convey a Hazard to the Foetus.

Many drugs used to treat maternal conditions in pregnancy convey a small − usually very small − risk to the foetus. The use of these agents depends on judgement of a balanced risk. That is, if the maternal condition was left untreated, the risk to mother and foetus would be greater than any potential hazard of the treatment to the foetus.

Fortunately, with most of these agents, the chance of harm to the foetus can be reduced to a minimum if the choice of drug is appropriate and it is used correctly.

Whether or not the patient is informed of any small chance of foetal damage is a matter for the judgement of the obstetrician. He may feel that the anxiety created by informing the patient would be such that she should not be told of some remote adverse possibility, particularly if she is already aware that her medical condition is of itself an added risk. In these circumstances many obstetricians would feel ethically justified in not alarming the patient unnecessarily.

ANAESTHETICS

Any ill-effect of general anaesthesia on the foetus is probably related to anoxia; if severe or prolonged maternal anoxia is avoided there should be no risk. The status of the foetus may be affected by the use of unnecessarily large doses of short-acting barbiturates used for induction of anaesthesia for elective caesarean section (Holdcroft et al., 1974).

Foetal methaemoglobinaemia may follow the use of prilocaine given for continuous epidural anaesthesia (Climie et al., 1967); bupivacaine is the agent of choice.

ANALGESICS

There is very little evidence that aspirin or other salicylates are teratogenic or a cause of perinatal loss or reduced birth weight in humans. Large amounts of aspirin taken in late pregnancy by the mother may occasionally affect platelet function and factor XII levels and cause bleeding or petechiae in the foetus, and unnecessary use of salicylates should be discouraged.

Narcotics given to the mother may reduce intra-uterine activity of the foetus and cause respiratory depression in the newborn. The newborn may suffer from a withdrawal syndrome of apnoeic attacks, tachycardia hypotonia and hypothermia, and the babies of patients who have received narcotics require observation in a newborn intensive care unit for some days.

ANTIBIOTICS

There is a small risk of ototoxicity to the foetus of large doses of amino-glycoside antibiotics such as gentamicin, kanamycin, neomycin, streptomycin or tobramycin that are used in pregnancy. Where possible, alternative antibiotics should be employed. When an aminoglycoside is really necessary, then concentrations in maternal blood should be monitored to avoid excessive levels.

There are theoretical risks of foetal bone marrow depression or of the 'grey syndrome' of hypothermia and cardio-respiratory failure of the newborn, if chloramphenicol is used in late pregnancy. This antibiotic is rarely essential and it should be avoided.

Novobiocin used in late pregnancy can inactivate bilirubin binding sites in the newborn and lead to neonatal jaundice and even kernicterus. It should not be used in late pregnancy as alternatives are nearly always available. Long-acting sulphonamide preparations in late pregnancy have been found to have a similar risk. They should not be used in pregnancy, as there is some animal work suggesting that they might be teratogenic, and short-acting sulphonamides are preferable.

ANTICOAGULANTS

Dicoumarol is slow acting and difficult to control; this magnifies the risks of ante-partum haemorrhage, placental separation in labour and haematoma or haemorrhage in the newborn. Phenindione has similar risks but is a reasonable drug to use if haematological control is good. Warfarin therapy in the first trimester is known to have a small risk of causing epiphyseal damage and consequent skeletal deformities in the foetus. There is also a risk of growth retardation, mental retardation and connective tissue disorders in the foetus if warfarin is given in the first few weeks of pregnancy.

The use of anticoagulants in pregnancy should be restricted to patients where they are really necessary. In the first trimester, a continuous intravenous infusion of heparin, which does not pass the placenta, should be used for treatment of a serious deep vein thrombosis or a pulmonary embolus, reverting to subcutaneous heparin for prophylaxis. In the second trimester, warfarin is the easiest drug with which good control may be secured. In the last week or two of pregnancy, the patient is admitted to hospital and given intravenous heparin, which is stopped when labour is induced or starts spontaneously.

When a patient goes into labour whilst still taking a coumarin anticoagulant, the prothrombin level or 'thrombotest' result should be secured immediately. If the degree of anticoagulation is low or moderate, there is no need to take any action except to manage the third stage of labour correctly, with intravenous ergometrine, Brandt-Andrews removal of the placenta, and prompt manual exploration of the uterus if indicated. The baby is given vitamin K. If the degree of anticoagulation is high in early labour, the mother is given a small dose of vitamin K immediately. A full dose may create a hypercoagulable state just when the risk of thrombosis is greatest.

ANTIDEPRESSANTS

Lithium therapy is known to cause a proportion of babies to be born with cyanosis, lethargy, hypotonia, poor suckling, poor respiratory effort and, occasionally, congenital heart disease (Schou *et al.*, 1973). If lithium therapy is essential in pregnancy, maternal plasma lithium levels should be kept below 1 mmol/l.

Amphetamines may cause placental insufficiency and they may cause foetal thrombocytopenia, and their use in pregnancy is undesirable.

ANTI-EPILEPTIC DRUGS

Diazepam or barbiturates alone give a risk of sedative withdrawal syndromes in the newborn, requiring observation in a newborn care unit for at least two days after delivery. There is no clear evidence that either of these drugs are teratogenic. If an established epileptic can be managed on small doses of phenobarbitone alone during pregnancy, this may be the safest solution.

Phenytoin and probably also primidone convey a clear hazard of foetal abnormality, the overall risk being about 6 per cent, compared to 1 − 4 per cent in epileptics not taking the drugs (Smithells, 1976). Combinations of phenytoin with barbiturates may increase the risk; combination with carbamazepine may reduce it (Starreveld-Zimmerman *et al.*, 1974). Phenytoin interferes with folic acid absorption and this is its likely mode of teratogenic action. In the author's opinion it should not be given in pregnancy without folic acid supplements of ten mg daily by mouth. Some physicians feel that this may increase the risk of convulsions but in practice, if phenytoin dose is adequate, the risk is very small.

Ideally, the epileptic woman should be seen before she ever conceives. She can be started on folic acid supplements at that time and her anti-epileptic therapy adjusted in collaboration with a neurologist. Many mild epileptics will be found to be taking much larger doses of drugs than are really necessary. The folic acid supplements are then available at the time of greatest need, in the first few weeks of pregnancy, and control of the anti-epileptic drugs is usually easy, particularly if blood levels can be monitored.

At the present time, there is too little information about the newer anti-epileptic drugs given alone to make it clear whether or not they have the same risks as phenytoin.

ANTIMALARIALS

Abortion may result from quinine overdosage; foetal abnormalities have been thought to occur after large doses. Nonetheless, in countries where malaria is endemic and only quinine is freely available, it is safer to give quinine prophylaxis than to risk malarial attacks. Mepacrine or pyrimethamine given with folic acid have not been shown to affect the foetus and these drugs are preferable. Chloroquine in high doses has been thought to be associated with foetal cochlear and retinal damage. Though the numerical risk is small, the drug should be avoided in pregnancy where possible.

ANTIMITOTIC AGENTS (LOCAL)

There is a theoretical risk of teratogenesis with idoxuridine. The drug is relatively ineffective therapeutically in herpes genitalis, and symptomatic measures are preferable. Podophyllin has been thought to cause foetal loss (Chamberlain et al., 1972); perineal warts in pregnancy can be treated symptomatically or, if extensive, by cautery under anaesthesia.

ANTITHYROID DRUGS

Partial thyroidectomy should be considered before or even during pregnancy; this minimizes the need for drug therapy. Carbimazole, methimazole and thiouracil all pass the placenta and may cause foetal goitre and hypothyroidism. If the drugs must be used they should be combined with l-thyroxine, which may help to protect the foetus, though the evidence for this is open to question. Iodides may also cause foetal goitre. Many preparations for bronchitis and asthma contain iodides; they should not be used in pregnancy. Radioactive [129]I is short acting and relatively safe for investigations but it is better to free thyroxine index and use clinical assessments of thyroid status.

HYPOGLYCAEMIC DRUGS

In animals the oral hypoglycaemic drugs can be teratogenic but this has not been confirmed in humans. The preferred treatment for diabetes mellitus in pregnancy is diet and insulin. Chlorpropamide has been used successfully with a good foetal outcome, but the newborn may be hypoglycaemic (Zucker and Simon, 1968).

HYPOTENSIVE DRUGS

Ganglion-blocking drugs such as pentolinium cause a 50 per cent incidence of fatal neonatal hypotension and paralytic ileus and should not be used in pregnancy. Reserpine causes foetal bradycardia, upsets the newborn thermal control and causes nasal obstruction in the newborn; its use in pregnancy is undesirable. Thiazide diuretics can, rarely, give rise to newborn thrombocytopenic purpura; there is only a small place for their use in pregnancy; frusemide can cause maternal haemoconcentration and reduced placental perfusion.

Propranolol seems relatively harmless in mild and moderate hypertension (Eliahou et al.,1978) or in the control of arrhythmias or hypertrophic cardiomyopathy in pregnancy. It may prevent vasodilation in the utero-placental circulation and pass to the foetus, impairing autonomic responses. If used in large doses for severe hypertension, propranolol treatment is associated with a high perinatal mortality, particularly if therapy was initiated in pregnancy (Stirrat and Lieberman, 1977). Moderate doses of oxprenolol started early in the third trimester of pregnancy seem to do no harm.

Diazoxide is occasionally used as a single dose in pregnancy to control an acute hypertensive episode. With continuing use there is a risk of disturbance of hair formation in the foetus and the drug may also interfere with carbohydrate metabolism in the foetus. Hydrallazine seems to have no particular ill-effects on the foetus and may improve the utero-placental circulation (Johnson and Clayton, 1957) but maternal intolerance is common with prolonged use, the drug causing headaches and skin rashes. Guanethidine does not harm the foetus but its autonomic blocking effects may cause maternal problems in a complicated confinement. Newer hypotensive drugs such as clonidine or debrisoquine have not been adequately evaluated in pregnancy for their use to be recommended.

It is for these reasons that methyldopa has become the most widely used hypotensive drug in pregnancy. It is the only agent which has been clearly shown to improve the prognosis for the foetus in pregnancies complicated by essential hypertension (Leather et al., 1968; Redman et al., 1976). Methyldopa sometimes causes a positive Coombs' test in the newborn but haemolytic anaemia has not been recorded. Very large doses (more than 2 g/day) have been thought to cause meconium ileus in the newborn (Clark et al., 1972), but this is rare.

Ideally, essential hypertension should be controlled with methyldopa before the patient ever conceives. If absolutely necessary small doses of propranolol or a diuretic may be included in the regimen. During pregnancy control is maintained by increasing doses as necessary, with hospital rest, by using hydrallazine to deal with acute exacerbations, and in late pregnancy, by delivering the baby.

IMMUNOSUPPRESSIVES

Hundreds of patients with cadaver renal transplant have now gone through pregnancy taking azathioprine as well as steroids. The incidence of obstetric complications is high in some, but not all, series; there seems to be no increase in foetal abnormality. A risk is virus infection, either cytomegalovirus or herpes genitalis. Cervical swabs should be cultured for virus at intervals and elective caesarean section considered if the cervix is infected when delivery is contemplated.

SEX HORMONES

Androgens have been used in the hope of preventing habitual abortion. They may cause masculinization of a female foetus and they are ineffective therapeutically.

Stilboestrol was widely used at one time in high risk pregnancies, both in America and in Europe. Continued use of the drug in pregnancy gives a risk that teenage female offspring will develop vaginal adenosis and perhaps vaginal adenocarcinoma (Poskanzer and Herbst, 1977). Most cases of adenocarcinoma were found in Boston and Chicago. Although the drug was widely used in Great Britain, only two cases had been reported (Monaghan and Sirisena, 1978). Stilboestrol is valueless as a therapeutic agent in pregnancy.

If progestagens are used in pregnancy, then a 17 α-hydroxy-steroid such as hydroxyprogesterone should be prescribed.

Hormone pregnancy tests consisting of a combination of oestrogen and progestagen, given in the hope of procuring withdrawal bleeding, have seldom been used by orthodox obstetricians, who employ urine tests for chorionic gonadotropin to confirm a diagnosis of pregnancy. Use of the oral tests has now been found to be associated with an increased incidence of foetal abnormality (Greenberg et al., 1977), and most of the preparations used have been withdrawn from the market. If a patient has taken such a test, the magnitude of the risk to her foetus is very small.

Pregnancies conceived whilst the patient is taking an oestrogen – progestagen oral contraceptive, or shortly after ceasing to take the contraceptive pill, have been found to be associated with a slightly increased chance of foetal abnormality (Janerich *et al.*, 1974). The defects vary in different reports, but the association is probably real. The magnitude of the risk, from the point of view of the individual patient, is extremely small. Nevertheless it is the author's practice to ask high risk patients to wait three months after ceasing to take an oral contraceptive before conception is permitted. This approach is easily justified by the advantage in managing an accurately dated pregnancy.

VITAMIN D

Patients taking high doses of calciferol, dihydrotachysterol or synthetic vitamin D derivatives during pregnancy, have a small risk of a baby with skeletal deformities. The risk is minimal if plasma calcium and phosphate levels are carefully monitored and balanced throughout pregnancy.

Agents Which Have Been Suspected of Teratogenicity, But For Which There Is No Good Evidence That They Are Harmful

It is very easy to accuse a drug on the basis of an isolated case or two, or because of a theoretical risk. It may take years of large-scale prospective studies to exonerate that drug. In the interim it is reasonable to use an alternative drug if one is available.

ANAESTHETIC GASES

There are studies which suggest that pregnant operating theatre personnel are at increased risk of abortion, but no clear evidence that the congenital abnormality incidence is higher than in control subjects (Knill-Jones *et at.*, 1972). It is likely that liability to abortion in operating theatre personnel is conditioned by the physical and psychological characteristics of the individuals concerned and the stresses to which they are subjected. It is therefore reasonable to advise such women, particularly if they are anxious or have a poor obstetric history, to seek more restful employment during their pregnancies (Hawkins and Love, 1978).

As a matter of general principle it is desirable that scavenger systems which reduce atmospheric contamination with anaesthetic gases should be installed in operating rooms.

ANTACIDS

Retrospective studies (Nelson and Forfar, 1971) have suggested an increased incidence of congenital abnormalities when antacids have been ingested during the first few weeks of pregnancy, but this has not been confirmed in prospective studies. As a matter of general principle, it is better to employ dietary measures and simple magnesium trisilicate mixtures in early pregnancy rather than newer agents containing local anaesthetics, belladonna alkaloids or drugs affecting gastric motility or acid secretion, whose potential ill-effects in pregnancy are really unknown.

ANTI-EMETICS

Nearly all anti-emetics have, at one time or another, been accused of teratogenicity. Extensive studies of several of the drugs have demonstrated these fears to be groundless. If the use of an anti-emetic is necessary, then preference should be given to promethazine or its theoclate, which have been very widely used for 25 years without being accused, and to pyridoxine, which is a natural vitamin.

ANTIMICROBIAL DRUGS

Cotrimoxazole has an anti-folic acid effect and the statement that it should not be used in pregnancy is often made, to protect the manufacturers. In fact it has been widely used in human pregnancy without apparent harm. The careful practitioner will give oral folic acid supplements if he prescribes cotrimoxazole in pregnancy. Short-acting sulphonamides pass the placenta and have been said to interfere with bilirubin conjugation in the foetus, rendering it liable to neonatal jaundice. The contraindication is to the use of sulphonamides prophylactically when premature labour is anticipated or in labour, particularly if there is Rhesus isoimmunization. Sulphonamides are also contraindicated in late pregnancy if the patient has glucose-6-phosphate dehydrogenase deficiency, when there is a risk of foetal methaemoglobinaemia.

Metronidazole has been widely used in human pregnancy and there is good evidence that it is not harmful (Morgan, 1978). There is no reason to withhold treatment with metronidazole for trichomoniasis in pregnancy, but on general principles it may be reasonable to defer treatment to the second trimester if the infection is asymptomatic.

INTRA-UTERINE CONTRACEPTIVE DEVICES CONTAINING COPPER

If pregnancy occurs with a device retained in the uterus, half the patients have a spontaneous abortion. Large-scale studies suggest no increase in congenital abnormalities if the pregnancy continues (Snowden, 1976).

IRON

Prospective studies have failed to confirm that iron taken in early pregnancy is harmful (Royal College of General Practitioners, 1975) but if haematinics are to be given prophylactically or for mild anaemia they can easily be deferred until the second trimester.

SEDATIVES AND TRANQUILLIZERS

There is a slightly increased incidence of minor foetal abnormalities in patients treated with barbiturate treatment in pregnancy, but the Royal College of General Practitioners (1975) were able to show that the association is not causal. Barbiturates are a common cause of skin rashes, which resolve with symptomatic measures when the drug is discontinued. Given in late pregnancy, barbiturates are thought to assist enzyme-induction in the foetus and thus aid the metabolism of bilirubin (Trolle, 1968).

Large doses of barbiturates given in labour can produce a newborn withdrawal syndrome (Desmond et al., 1972) and they should not be used in labour.

Meprobamate has been thought to be associated with an increase in foetal abnormality rate; monoamine oxidase inhibitors and tricyclic antidepressants might increase the vulnerability of the foetus to stress in labour. With all these agents the case is not proved.

STEROIDS

Large doses of glucocorticoid can cause foetal abnormalities, particularly cleft palate, in mice. Although the drugs have now been used to treat major medical disorders in pregnancy for 20 years, there is still no sound evidence that they predispose to foetal abnormality in humans, and fairly good evidence that they do not (Bongiovanni and

McPadden, 1960).

Previous use of oral contraception has been said to be associated with neonatal jaundice, but the evidence that the relationship is causal is unconvincing.

Drugs and Lactation

It is important to consider potential effects on lactation and the newborn when prescribing for the mother in the puerperium.

DRUGS WHICH MAY INHIBIT LACTATION

These are indicated in Table III. Alcohol, smoking, and fluid intake greater than 3 l/day, all act by inhibiting release of oxytocin from the posterior pituitary gland in the same way that they produce diuresis by inhibiting vasopression secretion. The stimulus to contraction of the myo-epithelial cells in the breast is thus impaired.

Table III
Drugs which may have the unwanted effect of inhibiting lactation

Alcohol in excess
Androgens
Atropine
Bromocryptine
Diuretics
Fluid intake in excess
Oestrogen-containing oral contraceptives
Smoking in excess

Androgens are sometimes still used in the United States of America to suppress lactation. Oestrogens are no longer used to suppress lactation in Great Britain owing to the increase in plasma coagulation factors they cause in some women and the associated risk of thrombosis or embolism. A combined oral contraceptive contains enough oestrogen to interfere with milk production in some women. If oral contraception is to be instituted whilst lactation continues, the risk of ovulation and conception is small and a low dose continuous progestagen preparation should be used until lactation ceases.

Bromocryptine, used to treat pituitary tumours, may be required in the mother's interests in the puerperium and this will suppress lactation by inhibiting prolactin secretion. In general, 'natural suppression'

— avoidance of stimuli to the breasts and analgesia where necessary — is used in Great Britain when lactation is not desired, but bromocriptine is sometimes used for suppression.

DRUGS WHICH HAVE TOXIC EFFECTS ON A BREAST-FED BABY

The only group of drugs which are necessary to the mother which absolutely contraindicate breast feeding are the antithyroid drugs. Potassium iodide can cause nodular goitre in the baby; thiouracil derivatives and carbimazole are actively secreted in breast milk and can cause goitre and cretinism in the baby and a small risk of agranulocytosis. Radioactive iodine can inhibit the newborn thyroid development and it is suspected that it might predispose to development of thyroid cancer in the child. Breast feeding should be suspended until the radioactive iodine has all been excreted if it is absolutely necessary for a thyroid function test.

Other drugs which may pass into breast milk to some degree are listed in Table IV. These agents should be used with caution in the nursing mother and the baby closely observed for ill-effects. Either the drug or the breast-feeding can be discontinued if necessary.

Table IV
Some drugs given to nursing mothers which might affect the breast fed baby

Drug	Suspected risk
Alcohol in excess	Neonatal drowsiness
Antibiotics	
Ampicillin, amoxycillin	Candidiasis (use oral nystatin prophylactically)
Benzylpenicillin	Very rarely, penicillin hypersensitivity
Cotrimoxazole, cotrimazine	Folic acid deficiency anaemia (check neonatal haemoglobin)
Gentamicin (large doses)	Ototoxicity
Nalidixic acid	Rarely, haemolytic anaemia
Streptomycin (large doses)	Ototoxicity
Sulphonamides (soluble)	Neonatal jaundice, if bilirubin conjugation inadequate
Tetracycline	Small risk of teeth discoloration
Anticoagulant	
Phenindione	Bleeding; use warfarin or give vitamin K supplements
Anticonvulsants	
Barbiturates (large doses)	Neonatal drowsiness
Phenytoin	Methaemoglobinaemia (rarely)
Primidone	Neonatal drowsiness

Table IV cont.

Drug	Suspected risk
Antidepressant	
Lithium	Hypotonia; neonatal plasma level half that of mother
Antithyroid drugs	
Carbimazole	Nodular goitre; cretinism
Iodides	Nodular goitre
Thiouracil	Nodular goitre; rarely, agranulocytosis
Aspirin in high dose	Bleeding tendency due to impaired platelet function
Atropine	Neonatal atropine effects
Fluoride (greater than 1 p.p.m. in water)	Mottling of teeth
Hypoglycaemics	
Tolbutamide	Hypoglycaemia
Hypotensive agent	
Propranolol	Beta-sympatholytic effects; hypoglycaemia
Laxatives	
Aloes	
Cascara	Purgation
Danthron	
Senna	
Oestrogens and oestrogen-containing oral contraceptives	Gynaecomastia in males. Precocious menstruation
Radioactive Iodine	Inhibits thyroid development; may predispose to thyroid cancer
Tranquillizers	
Chlorpromazine	Drowsiness; galactorrhoea
Diazepam	Drowsiness; weight loss; hyperbilirubinaemia
Vitamin D	
Calciferol (high doses)	Hypercalcaemia
Dihydrotachysterol	

Conclusion

Reduction in the incidence of congenital abnormalities and the production of healthy babies for those who desire them is not to be achieved by emotional over-reaction and withholding of necessary medicines during pregnancy and lactation, but by cautious and knowledgeable application of drug therapy only where it is really indicated. The practitioner who restricts his prescribing in pregnancy to well-established and widely used remedies which have been available for many years is unlikely to be responsible for foetal abnormalities.

References

Abortion Act (1967) London: HMSO.

Association of the British Pharmaceutical Industry (1980). *Data Sheet Compendium.* London: Datapharm.

Bithell, J.F., Draper, G.J. and Gorbach, P.D. (1973). Association between malignant disease in children and maternal virus infections. *British Medical Journal*, i, 706–708.

Bongiovanni, A.M. and McPadden, A.J. (1960). Steroids during pregnancy and possible fetal consequences. *Fertility and Sterility*, 11, 181–186.

British Medical Journal. (1972). Editorial. Neonatal behaviour and maternal barbiturates. *British Medical Journal*, iv, 63–64.

British Medical Journal. (1979). Editorial. Product liability. *British Medical Journal*, i, 1663–1664.

Butler, N.R., Goldstein, H. and Ross, E.M. (1972). Cigarette smoking in pregnancy: its influence on birth weight and perinatal mortality. *British Medical Journal*, ii, 127–130.

Chamberlain, M.J., Reynolds, A.L., and Yeoman, W.B. (1972). Toxic effect of podophyllum application in pregnancy. *British Medical Journal*, iii, 391–392.

Clark, A.D., Sevitt, L.H. and Hawkins, D.F. (1972). Use of frusemide in severe toxaemia of pregnancy. *Lancet*, i, 35–36.

Climie, C.R., McLean, S., Starmer, G.A. and Thomas, J. (1967). Methaemoglobinaemia in mother and foetus following continuous epidural analgesia with prilocaine. *British Journal of Anaesthesia*, 39, 155–159.

Committee on the Review of Medicines. (1979). Recommendations on barbiturate preparations. *British Medical Journal*, ii, 719–720.

Congenital Disabilities (Civil Liability) Act. (1976). London: HMSO.

Corbett, T.H., Cornell, R.G., Endres, J.L. and Lieding, K. (1974). Birth defects among children of nurse-anesthetists. *Anesthesiology*, 41, 341–344.

Court Brown, W.M., Doll, R., Spiers, F.W., Duffy, B.J. and McHugh, M.J. (1960). Geographical variation in leukaemia mortality in relation to background radiation and other factors. *British Medical Journal*, i, 1753–1759.

Davies, J.M., Latto, I.P., Jones, J.G., Veale, A. and Wardrop, C.A.P. (1979). Effects of stopping smoking for 48 hours on oxygen availability from the blood: a study on pregnant women. *British Medical Journal*, ii, 355–356.

Desmond, M.M., Schwanecke, R.P., Wilson, G.S., Yasanuga, S. and Burgdorff, I. (1972). Maternal barbiturate utilization and neonatal withdrawal symptomatology. *Journal of Pediatrics*, 80, 190–197.

Dewhurst, J., Ferriera, H.P., Dalley, V.M. and Staffurth, J.F. (1980). Stilboestrol-associated vaginal carcinoma treated by radiotherapy. *Journal of Obstetrics and Gynaecology*, 1, 63–64.

Donovan, J.W. (1977). Randomised controlled trial of anti-smoking advice in pregnancy. *British Journal of Preventive and Social Medicine*, 31, 6–12.

Eliahou, H.E., Silverberg, D.S., Reisin, E., Romem, I., Mashiach, S. and Serr, D.M. (1978). Propranolol for the treatment of hypertension in pregnancy. *British Journal of Obstetrics and Gynaecology*, 85, 431–436.

Fedrick, J. and Alberman, E.D. (1972). Reported influenza on pregnancy and subsequent cancer in the child. *British Medical Journal*, ii, 485–488.

Greenberg, G., Inman, W.H.W., Weatherall, J.A.C., Adelstein, A.M. and Haskey, J.C. (1977). Maternal drug histories and congenital abnormalities. *British Medical Journal*, ii, 853–856.

Hakulinen, T., Hovi, L., Karkinen-Jaaskelainen, M., Penttinen, K. and Saxen, L. (1973). Association between influenza during pregnancy and childhood leukaemia. *British Medical Journal*, iv, 265–267.

Hawkins, D.F. (1959). Birth weight and maternal smoking. *British Medical Journal*, ii, 820.

Hawkins, D.F. (1974). Habitual abortion. In *Obstetric Therapeutics*, edited by D.F. Hawkins, pp. 134–141. London: Baillière-Tindall.

Hawkins, D.F. (1976). Teratogens in the human: current problems. *Journal of Clinical Pathology*, **29**, Supplement 10, 150–156.

Hawkins, D.F. and Love, W. (1978). Counselling on the hazards of pregnancy in operating theatre staff. *Anaesthesia*, **33**, 96–97.

Holdcroft, A., Robinson, M.J., Gordon, H. and Whitwam, J.G. (1974). Comparison of two induction doses of methohexitone on infants delivered by caesarean section. *British Medical Journal*, ii, 472–475.

Holmberg, P.C. (1979). Central-nervous-system defects in children born to mothers exposed to organic solvents during pregnancy. *Lancet*, ii, 177–179.

Janerich, D.T., Piper, J.M. and Glebatis, D.M. (1974). Oral contraceptives and congenital limb-reduction defects. *New England Journal of Medicine*, **291**, 697–700.

Johnson, T. and Clayton, C.G. (1957). Diffusion of radioactive sodium in normal and pre-eclamptic pregnancies. *British Medical Journal*, i, 312–314.

Knill-Jones, R.P., Rodrigues, L.V., Moir, D.D. and Spence, A.A. (1972). Anaesthetic practice and pregnancy. Controlled survey of women anaesthetists in the United Kingdom. *Lancet*, i, 1326–1328.

Leather, H.M., Humphreys, D.M., Baker, P. and Chadd, M.A. (1968). A controlled trial of hypotensive agents in hypertension in pregnancy. *Lancet*, ii, 488–490.

Lenz, W. (1965). The chemistry and metabolism of thalidomide. In *A Symposium on Embryopathic Activity of Drugs*, edited by J.M. Robson, F.M. Sullivan and R.L. Smith, p. 182. London: Churchill.

McPherson, K., Smith, P. and Vessey, M.P. (1978). Teratogenic effects of waste anaesthetic gases. *British Medical Journal*, i, 437–438.

Magnin, P. (1962). L'avenir des enfants irradié *in utero*. *Presse Médicale*, **70**, 1199.

Medical Defence Union (1979). *Annual Report*, p. 24. London.

Merskey, E. and Rigal, W. (1956). Pregnancy in acute leukaemia treated with 6-mercaptopurine. *Lancet*, ii, 1268–1269.

Monaghan, J.M. and Sirisena, L.A.W. (1978). Stilboestrol and vaginal clear-cell adenocarcinoma syndrome. *British Medical Journal*, i, 1588–1590.

Morgan, I. (1978). Metronidazole treatment in pregnancy. *International Journal of Gynaecology and Obstetrics*, **15**, 501–502.

Naeye, R.L. (1978). Effects of maternal cigarette smoking on the fetus and placenta. *British Journal of Obstetrics and Gynaecology*, **85**, 732–737.

Nelson, M.M. and Forfar, J.O. (1971). Associations between drugs administered during pregnancy and congenital abnormalities of the fetus. *British Medical Journal*, i, 523–527.

Nora, A.H. and Nora, J.J. (1975). A syndrome of multiple congenital abnormalities associated with teratogenic exposure. *Archives of Environmental Health*, **30**, 17–21.

Ouellette, E.M., Rosett, H.L., Rosman, P. *et al.* (1977). Adverse effects on offspring of maternal alcohol abuse during pregnancy. *New England Journal of Medicine*, **297**, 528–530.

Poskanzer, D.C. and Herbst, A.L. (1977). Epidemiology of vaginal adenosis and adenocarcinoma associated with exposure to stilboestrol *in utero*. *Cancer*, **39**, 1892–1895.

Ravenna, P. and Stein, P.J. (1963). Acute monocytic leukaemia in pregnancy. *American Journal of Obstetrics and Gynecology*, **85**, 545–548.

Redman, C.W.G., Beilin, L.J., Bonnar, J. and Ounsted, M.K. (1976). Fetal outcome in trial of antihypertensive treatment in pregnancy. *Lancet*, **ii**, 753–756.

Royal College of General Practitioners (1975). Morbidity and drugs in pregnancy. *Journal of the Royal College of General Practitioners*, **25**, 631–645.

Schou, M., Goldfield, M.D., Weinstein, M.R. and Villeneuve, A. (1973). Lithium and pregnancy. I. Report from the register of lithium babies. *British Medical Journal*, **ii**, 135–136.

Smith, B.E. (1974). Teratology in anesthesia. *Clinical Obstetrics and Gynecology*, **17**, 145–163.

Smithells, R.S. (1976). Environmental teratogens of man. *British Medical Bulletin*, **32**, 27–33.

Snowden, A.R. (1976). IUCD and congenital malformation. *British Medical Journal*, **i**, 770.

Speidel, B.D. and Meadow, S.R. (1972). Maternal epilepsy and abnormalities of the fetus and newborn. *Lancet*, **ii**, 839–843.

Starreveld-Zimmerman, A.A.E., van der Kolk, W.J. and Meinardi, H. (1974). Teratogenicity of anti-epileptic drugs. *Clinical Neurology and Neurosurgery*, **77**, 81–95.

Sternberg, J. (1973). Radiation risk in pregnancy. *Clinical Obstetrics and Gynecology*, **16**, 235–278.

Stewart, A., Webb, J., and Hewitt, B. (1958). A survey of childhood malignancies. *British Medical Journal*, **i**, 1495–1508.

Stirrat, G.M. and Lieberman, B.A. (1977). Fetal outcome in pregnancies complicated by severe hypertension treated with propranolol. In *Therapeutic Problems in Pregnancy*, edited by P.J. Lewis, pp. 45–51. Lancaster: MTP Press.

Tomlin, P.J. (1979). Health problems of anaesthetists and their families in the West Midlands. *British Medical Journal*, **i**, 779–784.

Trolle, D. (1968). Phenobarbitone and neonatal icterus. *Lancet*, **i**, 251–252.

Tuchmann-Duplessis, H. (1965). Design and interpretation of teratogenic tests. In *A Symposium on Embryopathic Activity of Drugs*, edited by J.M. Robson, F.M. Sullivan and R.L. Smith, pp. 56–87. London: Churchill.

Vessey, M.P. (1979). Health problems of anaesthetists and their families. *British Medical Journal*, **i**, 1078–1079.

Wilkins, L. (1960). Masculinization of female fetus due to use of orally given progestins. *Journal of the American Medical Association*, **172**, 1028–1032.

Yerushalmy, J. (1971). The relationship of parents' cigarette smoking to outcome of pregnancy — implications as to the problem of inferring causation from observed associations. *American Journal of Epidemiology*, **93**, 443–456.

Zucker, P. and Simon, G. (1968). Prolonged symptomatic neonatal hypoglycaemia associated with maternal chlorpropamide therapy. *Pediatrics*, **42**, 824–825.

The Present Status of AID in the United Kingdom

J.R. NEWTON

*Department of Obstetrics and Gynaecology, University of Birmingham,
Birmingham, England*

Artificial insemination with donor semen AID has now produced more than 10 000 children world-wide, and we believe from the results of the Royal College of Obstetricians Survey that there are now more than 2000 women in the British Isles who are receiving this type of treatment from more than 40 clinics. These clinics are now scattered geographically throughout the British Isles and, following the Symposium in 1976 on artificial insemination, a co-ordinating committee was set up by the Royal College to assist these clinics in the collection of data, preparation of patient information documents and the standardization of the consent form.

Legal Issues Relating to AID

There are four main issues – these being: (1) Is AID legal without the husband's consent? (2) What is the status of the resultant child? (3) What is the liability of the doctor who carries out this type of procedure? (4) Should the origin of the child be disclosed to a third party? The last, of course, mainly relates to the registration of the birth of the child.

Cusine in his excellent paper in 1976 made it clear that the law has already decided that AID does not amount to intercourse (the case of McLennan v. McLennan 1958) and it is, therefore, not adultery for a wife to obtain AID without her husband's consent. This view, however, has not always been taken in other jurisdictions but probably this point is now academic since the alteration in the Divorce Reform Act 1969 and a similar Act in Scotland in 1976. These two Acts allow for divorce on grounds of irretrievable breakdown of marriage and, as part of this, intolerable conduct by the wife would obviously amount to irretrievable breakdown. It would be foolish, I think, for a doctor to undertake to carry out AID without the consent of the husband as this would amount to intolerable conduct.

Status of the Resultant Child

This does not appear to have been raised in any English Court. Legally, however, there does not appear to be much doubt about the status of the child born by AID. A child has the status of a legitimate child, if, and only if, it is born to or conceived by, or presumed to have been conceived by a couple during the substance of a valid marriage. The child born as a result of AID does not fulfil these requirements and is, therefore, illegitimate. This position has been reinforced by various authorities over the last twenty-five years and appears in most of the legal text books. Some people have tried to argue that because AID does not amount to adultery, the resultant child is legitimate. The reasoning, however, is fallacious because adultery is only one way of providing that the child was not conceived by the husband's sperm. The correct test is to ask what evidence is there to meet the requirements for the status of legitimacy, and in an AID situation this is clearly not the case. However, although the AID child does not fulfil the strict legal definition of legitimacy, it is I think correct to consider whether the child could be considered to be a legitimate child. It appears to be illogical and probably morally indefensible to discriminate between a child born by AID, a child conceived in adultery, or a child born to a single woman. To give an AID child the status of a legitimate child would mean creating a special status for that particular child. However, status is conferred by law and is independent of the volition of the individual, as for example in the case of an illegitimate child who subsequently becomes legitimate, or where the status of the legitimated child is conferred upon that child by the subsequent legally valid marriage of his parents if the parent was single beforehand, or the status of the adopted child is conferred by the judgement of a competent Court. Thus under the present rules an AID child cannot be given status of legitimacy. Before a child can be adopted it has to be at least 4½ months old and the consent of the natural parents has to be obtained. Despite this time problem it is possible for an AID child to be adopted by the parents.

A preferable approach would be to abolish the present status of legitimacy and to encompass in a single status all these problems, namely, that of the child in a single parent family or in the single parent family where the parent subsequently marries, a child that is adopted and the AID child. By changing the status of legitimacy to that of the accepted child, this would cover all categories and requires a simple change in the law governing the registration of births.

Liability of the Doctor

The third legal issue is the relationship between the doctor and the patients. Firstly, as regards the consents that are required, obviously these must be informed. Since the Symposium in 1976 on artificial insemination a patient document containing relevant information about artificial insemination, together with a consent form (which must be signed, witnessed and kept with the patient document so it is clear what the patient has been told) is now widely used in this country. This, together with the frank and full discussions by people trained in AID counselling leads one to believe that the majority of patients in this country indeed give informed consent. The second part of liability is, of course, the standards of skill required of the doctor in selecting suitable donors. The standard of care expected from a doctor in this case is that of reasonable competence, but this is a variable standard as has been reported in various textbooks on law, but it seems unlikely that the doctors in this country trained in AID counselling and having information to hand as to the rules and regulations concerning the selection of patients and donors, could possibly be called to task in a case of negligence. However, I think it necessary to look at the way in which donors are selected, as the practice seems to vary. For example, it is important that a full check of physical health is carried out, and that a test sample of semen is shown to be normal and free from infection, but it is also important to check on the donor's mental health and family background including the mental health of his parents and grand-parents. It is still unclear how far individual clinics go in matching the husband's physical characteristics, the colour of his hair, the stature and blood group. How many clinics carry out genetic tests, and what tests are these? There are still differences with regard to the intensity of donor screening and I think that this is one point in which minimal require-ments have to be set down, for to insist on a battery of intolerable investi-gations would turn away potential donors. However, until there is a test case, it is not possible to say what the minimal requirements are, but perhaps an analogy can be drawn from the standards of care expected from the donation of other biological material, for instance, blood. The British Medical Association (BMA) panel on human AID in 1973 stated that the selection of donors of semen requires care and attention, and emphasized that a most thorough examination of prospective donors should be undertaken before they are asked to give specimens. As far as the minimal requirements are concerned in my own clinic, these are: a full medical history, a family history with particular attention to any form of inherited hormone disease or mental disease, a simple physical examination, a check of blood group and karyotype and a test sample of sperm. This last is checked carefully for morphology, for other criteria of normality, for the presence of bacteria. This sample is then test frozen to make sure there are no problems with freezing.

The doctor's liability to the unborn child may at one time have been a matter of conjecture, but the Congenital Disabilities (Civil Liability) Act 1976 clearly gives the right of action to a child who is born incapacitated as the result of an occurrence before its birth. Such an occurrence is one which affected either parent of the child in his or her ability to have a normal healthy child, or affected the mother during her pregnancy, or affected her or the child in the course of its birth so the child is born with disabilities which would not have otherwise been present. It is, therefore, clear that the doctor could be sued on behalf of a child that is born defective if the doctor is negligent in relation to the selection of a donor. So far there have been no test cases in this country and, provided that adequate selection of donors takes place, it is unlikely that an action could ever be brought successfully.

Disclosure of Child's Origins at the Registration of Birth

The statutes dealing with registrations of births specify the particulars to be entered in the register. The 1953 and 1965 Acts specify the name and status of the mother and the father if the latter is known. Because the AID child is illegitimate, father unknown should be entered in the register, but it is widely accepted that some degree of falsification takes place and is probably inevitable. When the situation is explained to patients in clinical practice, the majority do not wish to involve in any way the third party in the identification of what they consider to be a highly confidential type of medical treatment. Because they wish to keep the matter secret they then are forced into a situation where falsification of the birth register almost certainly takes place. I cannot remember the last couple who decided for legal reasons to insist that their AID child was adopted, and I suspect that there are very few recorded cases. It is clear that at present this state of affairs is unnecessary and potentially harmful to sensible parents who are forced unnecessarily into making a ridiculous decision. It is imperative that we seek help and advice to change the status of the AID child to that of accepted child, for this would remove the problem. Likewise, unlike adoption, the child generally will not know that he is an AID child. In the last ten years I have only had one couple who have insisted on disclosing to the child his origins, although whether they have subsequently done this, I do not know. It was interesting that in that one case, the mother herself was an adopted child, and had not found out until she was eighteen years of age. This discovery had completely shattered her relationship with her mother. However, it may be instructive to ask whether the AID child ought to be able to ascertain the identity of his father, and whether there are any situations where the donor's identity may be revealed despite the donor's wishes. However, during the discussions with prospective AID parents, the doctor agrees never to reveal the identity of the donor. If, however, any action were to be raised by an AID child, or by a third party on behalf of that child against the doctor suggesting that the latter was negligent, the doctor would probably be required to reveal the donor's identity in order to explain his actions, and to satisfy a Court of Law. In these situations it is often helpful if a second doctor has examined the patient, i.e. the donor, and carried out the tests, as this helps to strengthen the case against negligence. Cusine (1976) emphasizes the importance of this aspect.

Clinical Trials and Record Systems

INTRODUCTION

Since the first births were recorded following the use of frozen semen (Bunge *et al.*, 1954), several papers have described individual physicians' experiences and some results of special AID clinics. It is unfortunate that there have been no large prospective clinical trials to ascertain answers to such basic questions as whether fresh or frozen semen gives a higher conception rate, the volume of semen that should be used, and the best position for the patient. Only one collaborative review by Sherman (1973), describes the pooled data from fifteen physicians.

The Royal College of Obstetricians and Gynaecologists (RCOG) Study Group on artificial insemination (Newton, 1976), and the survey of AID clinics in 1977 has shown that there is a great need to collate the experience of this procedure in England which now may have more than 2500 patients under treatment.

Table I
Clinical results with AID

1954	Bunge, Keettel and Sherman	First pregnancy from stored spermatozoa
1964	Perloff, Steinberger and Sherman	Four births with nitrogen vapour technique.
1973	Sherman	First collated results, 500 births from AID
1973	Smith and Steinberger	Comparison of fresh and frozen semen
1975	Chong and Taymor	16-year survey of 186 patients, 77 pregnancies with AID
1976	Dixon and Buttram	Cervical cup for AID
1976	Schoysman and Deboeck	15-year survey 412 pregnancies with AID
1976	Klay	Clomiphene induction to synchronize ovulation for AID
1976	David and Avidan	Psychological aspects of AID
1976	RCOG Symposium on Artificial Insemination	
1977	Jackson and Richardson	40-year survey of AID, 418 pregnancies
1977	Friberg and Gemzell	103 pregnancies with AID. Fresh sperm if no success after 6 months
1977	Pennington and Naik	Pregnancy rate similar at each month of treatment
1978	Sulewski *et al.*	Influence of rest, position of patient, and cervical cup on success
1978	Bromwich *et al.*	Use of life table analysis for results
1979	RCOG Workshop on AID, use of frozen semen (Richardson *et al.*)	

REVIEW OF PUBLISHED WORK

Table I shows the key references and reviews on the clinical results of AID with both fresh and frozen semen from the early reports of successful pregnancies 1954−1978. More than 1800 births by AID have so far been reported and, of the current thirty to forty references per year on artificial insemination, some six to ten per year deal with clinical problems.

Table II summarizes the conception rate and results at three and six months of treatment, Table III the live births, miscarriage rate, incidence of foetal abnormalities and sex of child, and Table IV lists details of the insemination technique. The data are incomplete as some authors do not give full details of patient population, pregnancy rate or sex of child. However, from a review of these and other published work it is reasonable to comment on factors which might influence the overall success of the treatment.

PREGNANCY RATE; OVERALL SUCCESS AND RATE AT THREE AND SIX MONTHS

Only one publication (Bromwich *et al.*, 1978) presents results both in pregnancies per cycle of treatment and by cumulative life table analysis. Jackson and Richardson (1977) present their data as cumulative rates (as percentages) per cycle of treatment. The remaining clinical studies report on overall percentage success ranging from 22 per cent to 72 per cent. These figures can be misleading as they do not take into account anovular cycles, failure of the patient to attend for treatment and those 'lost to follow-up'. The success rates after three and six months of treatment have to be interpreted with caution due to these problems, and at three months vary widely from 36 per cent to 73 per cent and at six months from 62 per cent to 95 per cent. It would be surprising if this degree of variation is due to differences in techniques, as these appear similar (see Table IV).

Nevertheless, it would appear that the majority of conceptions occur within the first six months of treatment, and thereafter the pregnancy rate declines rapidly with few patients conceiving after twelve cycles of treatment. It is unclear whether fresh semen has a higher pregnancy rate than frozen semen as there has been no large-scale clinical trial; however, there is a tendency for the conception rate to be slightly higher with fresh semen.

Table II
Success rate (conceptions) with AID

Year	Author	No. of patients	No. of pregnancies	Pregnancy rate overall (%)	Proportion of total pregnancies achieved:	
					In first 3 months (%)	In first 6 months (%)
1954	Bunge, Keettel, Sherman	—	4[a]	—	—	—
1973	Sherman et al.	?	621[a]	—	—	—
1975	Chong and Taymor	142	103	72	73	95
1976	Schoysman and Deboeck	?	412	22	50	72
1973	Smith and Steinberger	?	71(36[a])	—	44	83
1976	Dixon and Buttram	171	61	36	72	93
1977	Jackson and Richardson	604	355	59	39·2	62·8
1977	Friberg and Gemzell	?	103[a]	—	67	?
1977	Pennington and Naik	86	38	44	?	?
1978	Sulewski et al.	114	45	37	—	90
1978	Bromwich et al.	214	82[a]	38	36·6	65

[a] Frozen semen.

Table III
Pregnancies, miscarriage and sex of child

Year	Author	Sperm	Miscarriage rate	Live births	Male	Female	Abnormal births	Remarks
1973	Sherman et al.	Frozen	50 (8%)	564	–	–	7 (1%)	
1973	Smith and Steinberger	Fresh	4	35	19	11	–	
		Frozen	7	36	17	12	–	
1975	Chong and Taymor	Fresh	19 (18·4%)	84	39	45	1	
1976	Schoysman and Deboeck	Frozen	26 (26·8%)	152	33	30	2	
		Fresh	11 (16·4%)	87	30	21	3	
1976	Dixon and Buttram	Fresh	12	61	33	30	0	
1977	Jackson and Richardson	Fresh	43 (15·7%)	273	)187[a]	)189[a]	)7 (2%)	[a] includes AIH births as well.
		Frozen	2	17	)	)	)	
1977	Friberg and Gemzell	Frozen	?	90	42	48	1	
1977	Pennington and Naik	Frozen	–	15	–	–		
		Fresh	–	21	–	–		
1978	Sulewski et al.	Fresh/Frozen	4[b]	45	10[b]	6[b]	1[b]	[b] Only on sample of 21 pregnancies
1978	Bromwich et al.	Frozen	12 (14·6%)	82	26	15	1	

Table IV
Method of insemination

Year	Author	Fresh/Frozen	Type of insemination	Volume (ml)	Number of AID per cycle	Position	Aids to timing
1973	Smith and Steinberger	Fresh/Frozen	Intra-cervical	0·5	2	Dorsal	
1975	Chong and Taymor	Fresh					
1976	Schoysman and Deboeck	Frozen/Fresh	Intra-cervical	0·5	2	Dorsal lithotomy	BBT, mucus
1976	Dixon and Buttram	Fresh					
1977	Jackson and Richardson	Fresh/Frozen	Intra-cervical (metal cannula)	0·5–1·0	2–3	Dorsal – buttocks raised	BBT, mucus
1977	Friberg and Gemzell	Frozen	Intra-cervical (tuberculin syringe)	0·5	Daily (up to 6)	Dorsal	Plasma progesterone
1977	Pennington and Naik	Frozen					
1978	Sulewski et al.	Fresh/Frozen	Intra-cervical (tuberculin syringe)	Not recorded 0·5		Dorsal lithotomy	BBT
1978	Bromwich et al.	Frozen	Intra-cervical	0·5	2	Dorsal	BBT, mucus
1978	Matthews et al.	Frozen	Intra-cervical	0·5	2	Dorsal	LH surge by RIA

PATIENT POPULATION

The age range, previous gynaecological pathology, previous gynaecological surgery and the type of infertility investigation, especially with
regard to testing of tubal patency, all vary widely within the published
work. However, Dixon and Buttram (1976) were able to demonstrate the
influence of age and previous gynaecological disease, conception rate
not decreasing with age but decreasing with pelvic pathology. Friedman
in 1977 also commented on the influence of additional factors
(dysmenorrhoea, pelvic pathology) affecting the pregnancy rate, while
Schoysman and Deboeck (1976) found a high incidence of pelvic
pathology in patients who did not conceive after six cycles of treatment
and subsequently had laparoscopy and tubal patency tests.

INDICATIONS FOR REFERRAL

The majority of couples referred for treatment either had azoospermia
or oligospermia. The definition of oligospermia is not standardized but
appears in these series to be less than 10 – 30 million sperm per ml of
seminal fluid. Some oligospermic men had attempted AIH before being
referred for AID. Other causes for referral are listed as genetic, rhesus
disease, paraplegia and retrograde ejaculation.

With the inherent problems of variability in semen quality it is
essential that all men referred for AID shall have been adequately
examined and have had at least two seminal fluid analyses and, if
possible, a plasma FSH estimation. Despite this some people are still
referred without a definitive diagnosis (Newton, 1976).

LIVE BIRTHS, STILL BIRTHS, NEONATAL DEATHS

The outcome of pregnancy following AID with fresh or frozen sperm is
reassuring. The majority end in live births, and the rate of stillbirths,
due to obstetric or allied cause, and neonatal deaths does not appear to
be higher than after normal conception. However, a collaborative study
in England is needed to confirm this impression.

MISCARRIAGE RATE

First trimester miscarriages do occur after AID treatment and it is
unclear whether the rate is different from that occurring with normal
conception and whether there is any difference in the rate seen with
frozen or fresh semen. The overall rates vary from 8 to 27 per cent, and
there does not appear to be a trend either way with the use of frozen
semen.

FOETAL ABNORMALITIES

The individual series are small and it is not possible to draw conclusions from the foetal abnormality rate, except to say that the numbers of abnormalities are low and the use of frozen semen has not produced any startling increase. If anything, the rate may be lower with frozen semen than with fresh samples.

SEX OF CHILD

Here again the individual series are small, however pooled data do not suggest a bias towards either sex with this procedure. Relevant factors may be the length of survival of previously frozen sperm in the genital tract, the time of insemination relative to ovulation and the frequency of insemination.

FRESH VERSUS FROZEN SEMEN

From a practical point of view a daily clinic for AID will need to use frozen semen, as fresh samples may not be available every day. Three authors use both methods, Jackson and Richardson (1977), Schoysman and Deboeck (1976), Pennington and Naik (1977), while two others consistently prefer fresh semen, and the rest use frozen samples. Only one published trial of comparison between the two types of samples has been carried out (Smith and Steinberger, 1973). This was a small series and the results indicate small changes between the two in relation to conception rate, while no change was seen in the cumulative pregnancy rate at the end of six months.

However, Friberg and Gemzell (1977) suggest that if after six months of treatment with frozen semen no conception has occurred, then the patient should receive treatment with fresh semen.

METHOD OF INSEMINATION

The majority of authors cite intra-cervical insemination as their method of choice. Some however bathe the cervix with semen in addition and others inseminate small amounts into the uterine cavity. Bromwich *et al.* (1978) use a speculum to occlude the cervical canal to ensure correct insemination, while Chong and Taymor (1975) use a non-absorbable vaginal pack to prevent loss of the sperm samples after insemination.

The type of insemination cannula used varies from the curved metal cannula (Jackson and Richardson, 1977), the cervical cup (Sulewski *et al.*, 1978) and plastic cannula (Newton, 1976) for the fresh semen samples and thawed ampoule of frozen sperm. Those physicians using straws of frozen sperm use the straw attached to a syringe or insemination gun for direct insemination.

The majority of authors also take one drop of the sample for pre-insemination sperm analysis and some carry out a sperm invasion test on the recipient's mucus prior to AID.

POSITION OF PATIENT AND REST AFTER TREATMENT

Most employ either the dorsal or dorsolithotomy position for insemination. However, there is great variability in views on the need for rest after AID. One series (Sulewski et al., 1978) suggests that there is no need for rest after AID while others advocate rest for 10 to 30 minutes (Bromwich et al., 1978; Jackson and Richardson, 1977). Others suggest that in addition the buttocks need to be raised to prevent loss of the sample. There appear to be conflicting opinions which can only be resolved with large-scale trials.

TIMING OF AID

Probably due to the distance of the patient from the clinics and the lack of a seven day a week service, most authors rely on one or two inseminations per cycle. To aid the choice of day all use a menstrual calendar and basal body temperature chart, while three series assess mucus in addition. Friberg and Gemzell (1977) carried out daily insemination from day 11 of the cycle until the first significant rise of plasma progesterone, indicating that ovulation had occurred, while Matthews et al. (1978) used a rapid LH assay to pick up the mid-cycle surge to time insemination.

SYNCHRONIZATION OF OVULATION

Following the studies of Klay (1976) who used clomiphene to regulate and synchronize ovulation, many people have used ovulation induction to assist in the timing of AID. However, Schoysman and Deboeck (1976) showed there to be no difference in conception rates between stimulated and unstimulated (natural) cycles. There are suggestions in other work (Bromwich et al., 1978) that the conception rate may in fact be lower with clomiphene stimulation than with natural cycles.

While clomiphene is obviously important for use in irregular cycles or long cycles and with anovular patients, its use in the normal patient still has to be evaluated.

OTHER POINTS COVERED IN PUBLISHED WORK

Kaptetanakis *et al.* (1977) have reported the successful recovery of sperm with the modified voiding technique in ten cases of retrograde ejaculation. A fraction of these motile sperms were used for insemination and the rest stored frozen with good post freeze/thaw recovery rates. They report ten pregnancies with eight live births and two miscarriages.

Quinlivan (1978) reports on the prevalence of raised sperm agglutinating antibodies with wives of couples undergoing AID. This small series also suggests a lower pregnancy rate in this group who are also having normal intercourse as well as AID, compared with a different group advised to either abstain or use condoms over the time of AID and ovulation. This interesting point is worth further evaluation.

RCOG SURVEY 1977

In the autumn of 1977 the AI Sub-committee of the RCOG sent out a confidential questionnaire to 38 centres in the United Kingdom. Twenty-seven replied (71 per cent) and of them 22 (81.5 per cent of those returned) were already providing an AID service. Geographical distribution within the United Kingdom was uneven. Wales, the North-East, East Anglia and Southern England had no AID service at the end of 1977. The Midlands had only two centres but London had seven. The majority of centres had had difficulty in setting up a service, and this was usually due to lack of finance.

In 1977 approximately 2396 couples were referred for AID, 1200 were receiving treatment, and in the previous year 731 pregnancies had been achieved by AID.

There appeared to be no standard method of investigation of the couple prior to AID being started, and there was no standard method of examination and selection of donors. The majority of donors were students and most were reimbursed for the semen samples. Many centres used both fresh and frozen semen, the choice depending on availability, but the number of pregnancies achieved with fresh semen was higher than with frozen semen.

Most of the centres charged a fee for the service, although often the fee was nominal, and eight centres were stated to be NHS centres. The number of staff used to run the centre varied widely, and funding often came from several sources.

RECORD SYSTEMS

No standardized system is in operation, but whatever system is used complete confidentiality of both the donor and recipient is needed. Usually the initial discussion and decision to treat with AID is recorded in the patient's notes. However, the consent form and treatment sheet should be kept separately. It is important to record the clinical details of the patient on the treatment sheet, cross-referenced to the notes and also to include details of the husband's physical characteristics, diagnosis and blood group.

The clinical record sheet (Table V) should record the minimal data but individual clinics may wish to record additional data, e.g. hormone analysis results. At the end of each month of treatment it is recommended that the data be transcribed to Cope Chat punch cards or computer tape for future analysis recording the number and day of insemination, length of cycle, whether ovulation occurred and conception if any. Any additional treatment, for example oestrogen or fertility drugs needs to be recorded. For those who become pregnant records of the outcome of pregnancy need to be obtained.

For frozen semen samples, major problems of sample identification are present. Whichever method is chosen it needs to be simple to allow quick extraction of the semen sample without temperature change of the rest of the samples. This removal should take place within the nitrogen vapour phase if possible. Sample identification and localization will depend on the type of container, be they straws, ampoules or pellets. The donor code number and date of sample needs to be clearly marked on the sample and its position in the churn recorded in the sample storage ledger.

For straws the use of a self-adhesive label wound round one end of the straw as a flag prevents the straw falling through the bottom of the container, and in addition a colour code of straw (six colours) plus PVA filter (six colours) provides an additional safeguard. For ampoules the canes holding them can be colour coded and the donor code etched on to the ampoule with an electric pen.

The donor code book should be kept near to the storage churn and in it recorded basic details of the donor's characteristics: donor number, blood group, height, build, hair colour, and eye colour. A duplicate of this code is kept in the clinic record book to allow rapid selection of the appropriate sample.

Conclusions

There is a definite need for continuing clinical research into AID in this

Table V
Suggested treatment chart

AID number .... Name ....

Hospital number .... Address ....

                                        Telephone No. ....

Diagnosis .... Husband's characteristics: height, hair colour, eye
                                        colour, build

| Date | Day of cycle | Mucus Assessment | | | Donor code | Post thaw recovery | Other test | Remarks and results of treatment |
		SBK	Cells	Other				

country. Collaboration between centres which has started over the last two years following the RCOG workshop on artificial insemination should continue. If the various clinics could agree on common protocols for investigation and treatment, many of the unanswered questions posed in this review could be solved.

References

Bromwich, P., Kilpatrick, M. and Newton, J.R. (1978). Artificial insemination with frozen stored semen. *British Journal of Obstetrics and Gynaecology*, **85**, 641–644.

Bunge, R.G., Keettel, W.C. and Sherman, J.K. (1954). Clinical use of frozen semen: report of four cases. *Fertility and Sterility*, **5**, 520–529.

Chong, A.P. and Taymor, M.L. (1975). Sixteen years' experience with therapeutic donor insemination. *Fertility and Sterility*, **26**, 520–529.

Cusine, D.J. (1976). AID and the law. *Journal of Medical Ethics*, **1**, 39–41.

David, A. and Avidan, D. (1976). Artificial insemination donor: clinical and psychological aspects. *Fertility and Sterility*, **27**, 528–532.

Dixon, R.E. and Buttram, V.C. (1976). Artificial insemination using donor semen: a review of 171 cases. *Fertility and Sterility*, **27**, 130–134.

Friberg, J. and Gemzell, C. (1977). Sperm freezing and donor insemination. *International Journal of Fertility*, **22**, 148–154.

Jackson, M.C.N. and Richardson, D.W. (1977). The use of fresh and frozen semen in human artificial insemination. *Journal of Biosocial Science*, **9**, 251–262.

Klay, L.J. (1976). Clomiphene-regulated ovulation for donor artificial insemination. *Fertility and Sterility*, **27**, 383–388.

Matthews, C.D., Ferin, J.F.P., Hopkins, R., Wheatley, B.P., Makin, M. and Svigors, J.M. (1978). The characterization of thawed semen and the timing and route of insemination associated with conception in the human. *International Journal of Fertility*, **23**, 158–159.

Newton, J.R. (1976). Current status of artificial insemination in clinical practice. In *Artificial Insemination*, edited by M. Brudenell, A. McClaren, R. Short and M. Symonds. Proceedings of the Fourth Study Group of the Royal College of Obstetricians and Gynaecologists. London: Royal College of Obstetricians and Gynaecologists.

Pennington, G. and Naik, S. (1977). Donor insemination: report of a two-year study. *British Medical Journal*, i, 1327–1330.

Perloff, W.H., Steinberger, E. and Sherman, J.K. (1964). Conception with human spermatoza frozen by nitrogen vapor technique. *Fertility and Sterility*, **15**, 501–504.

Quinlivan, D. and Sullivan, H. (1978). Spermatozial antibodies in human seminal plasma as a cause of failed artificial donor insemination. *Fertility and Sterility*, **28**, 1082–1085.

Richardson, D., Joyce, D. and Symonds, M. (Editors) (1979). *Frozen Human Semen*. Proceedings of a workshop upon the cryobiology of human semen, and its role in Artificial Insemination by Donor, 1979. London: Royal College of Obstetricians and Gynaecologists.

Schoysman, R. and Deboeck, A. (1976). Results of donor insemination with frozen semen. Sperm action. *Progress in Reproductive Biology*, 1, 252.

Sherman, J.K. (1973). Synopsis of the use of frozen human semen since 1964: state of the art of human semen banking. *Fertility and Sterility*, 24, 397–412.

Smith, K.D. and Steinberger, E. (1973). Survival of spermatoza in a human sperm bank: effects of long-term storage. *Journal of the American Medical Association*, 223, 774–777.

Sulewski, J.M., Eisenberg, F. and Stenger, V.G. (1978). A longitudinal analysis of artificial insemination with donor semen. *Fertility and Sterility*, 29, 527–531.

Medical and Social Hazards of Teenage Pregnancy

J.K. RUSSELL

Department of Obstetrics and Gynaecology, University of Newcastle upon Tyne, England

Some Associations of Pregnancy in Young Schoolgirls

My clinical experience in obstetrics began in 1946 and I have been in practice constantly since that time. These thirty years have seen many changes, mostly for the better, but there have been some unwelcome developments — none more unwelcome or more distressing than the striking rise there has been in the number of pregnancies among young schoolgirls. In this chapter I will first, briefly, trace the measure of this increase using figures for England and Wales. Then in rather more detail and drawing from my own experience in Newcastle upon Tyne will present an account of some of the immediate and long-term problems faced by pregnant schoolgirls and their families. Throughout my presentation I will draw a distinction between schoolgirls aged 16 years and younger and older teenage girls aged 17 to 19 years. The medical and social problems faced by the two groups are rather different. The older girls, on the whole, are mentally and physically more mature, marriage is more of a possibility and reproductive efficiency is at its best in this age group.

The National Scene

In previous communications I have drawn attention to the striking rise in the number of pregnancies that took place in young teenagers from the late 1950s onwards. And to the disproportionate contribution young teenagers made from that time onwards to illegitimate pregnancy in England and Wales.

The 1967 Abortion Act has had the obvious and expected effect of arresting the dramatic rise in the number of completed pregnancies in

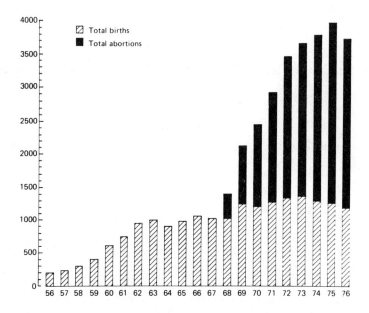

FIG. 1. Total births and therapeutic abortions per year in girls aged 15 years in England
and Wales (1956–1976).

young teenage girls, but the increase in the number of conceptions
continued unabated until very recently.

The Newcastle Scene

Drawing on my own clinical experience I should like to examine more
closely the meaning of these pregnancies for the young girls and for their
families.

Between September 1960 and September 1974 I was involved in the
management of 267 schoolgirls aged 16 years and under who were
referred to me at the Royal Victoria Infirmary or Princess Mary
Maternity Hospital with a first pregnancy. During the same period, at
the two hospitals, 317 single girls aged 17 to 19 years were referred with
first pregnancies. Circumstances in the North-East of England — a
fairly static population, the high standing of the two hospitals in the
community and a long history of close collaboration, for research
purposes, between the University, the Teaching Hospital and the

community health services — have helped me to maintain contact over the years with the majority of these girls and their families. I am especially indebted to family doctors, medical social workers and other professional colleagues for a great deal of follow-up information. In many instances I have dealt with the girls' subsequent pregnancies or gynaecological problems and from these various sources I am able to present in some detail the subsequent obstetric and personal histories of 238 of the young schoolgirls and 274 of the older teenagers, and to contrast their experiences. I have no reason to believe that the girls whose subsequent reproductive careers and personal histories I have been unable to check differ in any significant way from those who were traced. With very few exceptions the failure to obtain follow-up information was due to the girl having moved from the North East to another part of the country. The period of follow-up ranged from five to ten years.

Table I
Outcome of initial pregnancies

	16 years and under	17, 18, 19 years
Therapeutic abortion	167 (70%)	141 (51%)
Pregnancy continued	68 (28.5%)	128 (47%)
Spontaneous abortion	3	5
Totals	**238**	**274**

The outcome of the initial pregnancies is shown in Table I. Pregnancy was more often terminated in the younger girls.

The gestational age at first consultation is shown in Table II. The younger girls were twice as likely to appear after the twelfth week as the

Table II
Gestational age at first consultation

	7–10 weeks	10–12 weeks	13–16 weeks	Over 16 weeks	Total
16 years and under	45	112	51	30	238
17,18, 19 years	68	161	31	14	274

Table III
Technique of therapeutic abortions

	16 years and under	17, 18, 19 years
Hysterotomy	2	1
D and C	16	19
Prostaglandin	17	7
Suction	132	114
Total	**167**	**141**

older teenagers (35 per cent and 17 per cent).

The techniques used in termination are shown in Table III. The greater use of prostaglandin in the younger girls reflects the tendency for them to appear at a later gestational age.

Table IV
Immediate complications of therapeutic abortion

	16 years and under	17, 18, 19 years
Laceration of cervix requiring suture	9 (5·4%)	2 (1·4 %)
Blood transfusion at operation or within 24 h	4 (2·4%)	1 (0·7 %)
Retained products curettage in theatre	12 (7·2%)	3 (2·1 %)
Uterine infection requiring antibiotic therapy	10 (6%)	3 (2·1)%)

The next table lists the immediate complications and these were all demonstrably higher in the younger girls: a consequence, in my view, of

Table V
Outcome of pregnancies that continued beyond 28 weeks

16 yrs and under (68 pregnancies)	1 stillbirth : multiple deformation 1 neonatal death : 1800 g respiratory distress syndrome	2·9%

17, 18, 19 yrs (128 pregnancies)	1 stillbirth : cord round neck
	1 set of premature twins
	   1400 g : macerated
	   1200 g : pneumonitis
		2·3%

Table VI
Birthweight below 2500 grammes

	Number	%
16 years and under	6 out of 68	9
17, 18, 19 years	5 out of 128	3·9

the immaturity of the cervix and the greater risks attached to dilating the canal of the smaller cervix. Next, the outcome of the pregnancies that were allowed to continue in the two groups of girls. Table V reveals a perinatal mortality rate little, if at all, higher than that reported over the 15-year period.

Table VI records birthweight and does underline the matter of low birthweight in babies born alive to the young teenagers. In five out of six cases the low birthweight was due to premature onset of labour. During the 15-year period the incidence of low birthweight in England and Wales was around six to seven per cent.

Table VII
Pre-eclamptic toxaemia

	Number	Percentage
16 years and under	9 out of 68	13·2
17, 18, 19 years	11 out of 128	8·6
Princess Mary Maternity Hospital (1975)	329 out of 2819	11·7

Table VII gives the incidence of pre-eclampsia in the two groups and in the Princess Mary Maternity Hospital. A slightly increased incidence is noted in the young teenagers. The type of delivery in the two groups of teenagers is given in Table VIII, and these figures are remarkably similar to those for the whole hospital. (For example, during the period 1960 to 1969, the incidence of Caesarean section among primigravidae was 5 per cent and forceps delivery 17 per cent).

Table VIII
Type of delivery

	16 years and under		17, 18, 19 years	
	No.	%	No.	%
Spontaneous	52	74	100	78
Forceps	12	18	15	12
Caesarean section	2	4	9	7
Breech	2	4	4	3
Total	68		128	

In summary it has been my experience that these teenage girls, in their first pregnancies, do relatively well and pose few obstetric problems, probably the greatest being the risk of a low birthweight baby.

Table IX
133 Second pregnancies in 16 years and under whose first pregnancy was terminated

19 pregnancies terminated

114 continued : 24 aborted spontaneously (21%)
    (11 in first trimester; 13 in second trimester)

90 continued beyond 28 weeks :
    5 babies either stillborn or died in first week
    PMR — 55 per 1000

What of the pregnancies that followed these initial pregnancies? The following four tables record the outcome of the second pregnancies. First, those 167 young teenagers whose first pregnancy was terminated. One hundred and thirty-three have had a second pregnancy and I consider the spontaneous abortion and perinatal mortality rates to be significantly elevated (Table IX). All five babies who died were below 2500 g at birth. Next, the 68 young teenagers whose first pregnancy continued. Fifty-three have had a second pregnancy and their reproductive performance is noticeably better (Table X).

Table X
53 second pregnancies in 16 years and under whose first pregnancy continued

4 pregnancies terminated

49 continued : 4 aborted spontaneously (8%)
    (3 in first trimester; 1 in second trimester)

45 continued beyond 28 weeks :
    1 baby died in first week
    PMR — 22 per 1000

Of the 141 older teenage girls whose first pregnancy was terminated 102 have had a second pregnancy with a spontaneous abortion rate of 13 per cent and a perinatal mortality rate of 24 per 1000 (Table XI). Of the 128 older girls whose first pregnancy continued 101 have had second pregnancies with a spontaneous abortion rate of 6 per cent and a perinatal mortality rate of 21 per 1000 (Table XII).

These results point to a greater risk of an unsuccessful second pregnancy in the youngest girls if the first pregnancy is terminated by

Table XI
102 second pregnancies in 17, 18, 19 years whose first pregnancy was terminated

8 pregnancies terminated
94 continued: 12 aborted spontaneously (13%)
(9 in first trimester; 3 in second trimester)

82 continued beyond 28 weeks:
2 babies stillborn or died in first week
PMR — 24 per 1000

therapeutic abortion. The special hazards are spontaneous abortion or premature onset of labour.

Table XII
101 second pregnancies in 17, 18, 19 years whose first pregnancy continued

8 pregnancies terminated

93 continued: 6 aborted spontaneously (6%)
(4 in first trimester; 2 in second trimester)
87 continued beyond 28 weeks
2 stillbirths (twins at 30 weeks)
PMR — 21 per 1000

The following two tables (Tables XIII and XIV) list known social problems in the families of the two groups of girls. The likelihood of an obvious social problem is much greater in the families of the younger group of girls.

The educational implications were noticeably different in the two

Table XIII
Social Problems in the families of the 238 girls aged 16 years and under

	Years
Parents separated	39
Parents divorced	13
One or other parent known alcoholic	25
One or other parent in jail or been in jail	12
Close family history of illegitimacy	41
Child 'in care'	11
Child attending special school because of low IQ	9

Notes: Some cases are included under more than one heading but in 130 out of the 238 (55%) families there was an obvious social problem.

Table XIV
Social problems in the families of the 274 girls aged 17, 18 and 19 years

Parents separated	21
Parents divorced	9
One or other parent known alcoholic	12
One or other parent in jail or been in jail	7
Close family history of illegitimacy	23
History of girl having been 'in care' or having attended 'special school'	7

Note: Some cases are included under more than one heading but in 82 out of the 274 (29%) families there was an obvious social problem.

groups of girls. In the younger age group, when pregnancy was terminated, there was no single example of serious interference with the girls' educations. Among the 68 girls whose pregnancy continued there were 19 instances where the girl's education was either seriously interrupted or brought prematurely to an end. Again there was no recognized educational problem among the 141 older teenagers whose pregnancies were terminated and in only 11 of the 128 cases where pregnancy continued did the girls appear to suffer in an educational sense.

Many girls in each group were clearly anxious and concerned about the fact that they were pregnant but none, at the time of their first pregnancy, required active psychiatric support. But three of the younger and one of the older teenagers did run into serious psychiatric problems in later years — problems that were judged to be directly related to the first pregnancy. In three instances the abortion of the first pregnancy was later followed by a sequence of spontaneous abortions when the girl was married and wanted a family. This led, in each case, to severe depression that required psychiatric help. In the fourth case the girl had an acute depression followed by bouts of chronic depression when her husband discovered, after marriage, that she had had an illegitimate child at the age of 17 years. Apart from these four cases there were numerous other examples of marital tension, discord and unhappiness that were directly related by the girl to the first pregnancy before her marriage.

Four of the younger teenagers and three of the older age group have developed positive cervical smears during the period of the follow-up. I have dealt with each of them. Five have been managed conservatively and two have had modified radical hysterectomies having finished their families — one at the age of 26 years, the other at 28 years. In both cases there was extensive carcinoma *in situ* in the cervix.

SPECIAL CATEGORIES

Within these groups of pregnant, teenage girls is a small but important number who were either educationally subnormal or 'in care'. They invariably presented medical and social problems that were especially difficult to manage. In four cases where the girls' IQs were seriously subnormal the parents pressed very strongly for the child to be sterilized — three of the four pregnancies were claimed to have been fathered by boys themselves educationally subnormal. This emotive issue was fully and helpfully examined in a discussion paper sent by the Department of Health and Social Security (DHSS) to Regional and Area Health Authorities in October 1975. The intention, once responses had been received, was for the DHSS to issue a 'Code of Practice' in relation to the sterilization of children under the age of 16 years. The DHSS have since offered no firm guidelines and there the matter rests.

CONTRACEPTION

Particular attention was paid to the contraceptive needs of the girls in the younger age group. Of the 238 girls, 197 (83 per cent) admitted that they had either never used contraception or had sporadically used some form of contraception. Among the older teenagers the figure was 139 out of 274 (51 per cent). My suspicion is that a substantial number of the youngest teenage girls believed that they could not become pregnant either because they were too young or because they had intercourse too infrequently. I believe that the greatest deterrent to the effective use of contraception among the younger teenagers is the irregularity of intercourse. When intercourse is unanticipated, prevention of pregnancy is a considerable problem. Another difficulty is that the use of certain forms of contraception increases the risk that their sexual activity will be discovered by their parents — a matter that many of the girls put to me as an important consideration.

In spite of the best efforts of myself and my family planning colleagues at least 23 and probably a further nine of the original group of 238 young teenagers had unplanned and unwelcome pregnancies during the follow-up period.

Conclusions

The medical and social problems faced by pregnant teenagers aged 16 years and under are rather different from those faced by older teenagers.

In the face of an established pregnancy in the younger age group there is an obvious conflict between medical and social considerations. In my experience therapeutic abortion if requested — provided it is carried out within accepted gynaecological guidelines — is most likely to solve the immediate problem for the girl and her family but more likely to create problems in future childbearing. Continuation of a pregnancy at this early age, provided the child is well looked after, is not unduly worrying in the medical sense but is associated with considerable educational and social problems. There would seem to be fewer long-term effects on future reproduction.

Here — as with so many other medical problems — the special circumstances of each case have to be considered before a decision is made about management. It is not possible to state that there is a 'best line of management' in the face of pregnancy in young teenage schoolgirls.

Risks and Problems for the Older Parent

R.J. BEARD

Royal Sussex County Hospital, Brighton, Sussex, England

Parental age affects the ability to conceive, the pregnancy itself, the newborn child, and its later development. It is difficult always to separate the effects of parental age from those of social environment, intelligence, and particularly parity. As age advances, other diseases become more common, and these in turn can affect the pregnancy and its outcome. Today many older parents, or intending parents, as a result of newspaper and magazine articles or television and radio programmes, are aware that there may be problems, and they may seek advice concerning the advisability of trying for a child. It is therefore useful for the practitioner to be acquainted with the problems that can occur.

Incidence

Older parents today are giving birth to fewer children. Figure 1 shows the number of maternities by age in the years 1961 – 72, using data from the Department of Health and Social Security (1975), and there is a clear trend to reduction in older fertility. Since 1972 this trend has continued. For example, from 1965 to 1976 there was a fall from 28 per cent to 21 per cent in the number of women over the age of 30 who had babies, and from 3 per cent to 1·1 per cent for women over 40.

Further examination of the figures shows that it is the fertility of women with large families, and of those whose husbands were in the semi-skilled or unskilled occupations, that has fallen the fastest. Among those whose husbands were in professional or managerial posts, fertility has fallen the least, and this holds also for those of high parity in this class (Office of Population Censuses and Surveys, 1978a). Ninety per cent of women of Social Class V had had their first baby by the age of 25 and only 1 per cent after the age of 29. By contrast, only 45 per cent of Social Class I had had their first baby before the age of 25 and 13 per cent had their first baby after the age of 29 (Cartwright, 1976).

193

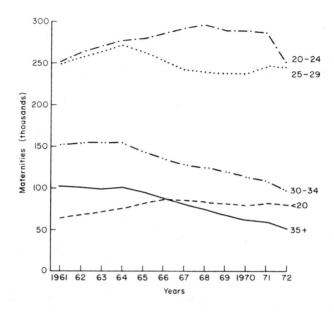

FIG. 1. Maternities (women having live or stillbirths) and notified abortions among women by age group (1961–1972).

This reduction in births is not matched by any reduction in the numbers of conceptions. A woman's ability to conceive does not fall significantly until a few years prior to the menopause, when the number of anovulatory cycles begins to increase and so reduces fertility. As the average age of the menopause in this country is about 51, the occurrence of pregnancy after 50 years of age is extremely unlikely. The steep decline in the number of deliveries in women aged 45 and over (Office of Population Censuses and Surveys, 1978a) is indicated in Fig. 2.

There has recently been a large increase in the number of older women requesting abortion, probably as a result of the many recent adverse reports about the effects of the combined oral contraceptive that have appeared in the lay press. For example, in the second quarter of 1978, whereas the overall increase in the abortion rate was 9·2 per cent, in the over 35 years-olds the increase was 17 per cent (Office of Population Censuses and Surveys, 1978b).

Pregnancy

Older women may find it less easy to be pregnant. They may have

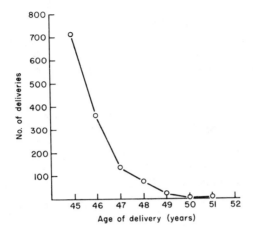

FIG. 2. Deliveries in women aged more than 44 years, England and Wales, 1967. Graphic representation of data from Registrar General's Statistical Review of England and Wales.

completed their intended family and many a late pregnancy is unwanted or at least unplanned. Despite the apparent increase in the number of abortion requests in this age group, most women of this age do not find it easy to take the decision to terminate a pregnancy. In a recent survey of women who were not themselves pregnant, 43 per cent of those over the age of 35 were against abortion, as compared with only 29 per cent under the age of 20 (Cartwright, 1976). Older women find the physical effort of being pregnant harder to sustain than when they were younger. Many feel themselves out of place in the antenatal clinic, where they are surrounded by women young enough to be their daughters. They may not be so keen to attend the antenatal classes, where their younger fellow participants are more agile, and where the older women may feel embarrassed at the difference.

When it is their first pregnancy, there may have been preceding infertility, and this heightens their anxiety. They feel isolated since they often have few friends of their own age who are similarly pregnant and with whom they can discuss events. Similarly, they are likely to have few friends with young children with whom they can communicate. Thus there is a tendency for them to become 'baby book minded'. Sometimes the knowledge they acquire causes more confusion and anxiety than is necessary. They are naturally worried about possible abnormality of the infant, and must be given more time in the consulting room to allow full discussion and explanation of the procedures for the prenatal diagnosis of Down's syndrome and neural tube defects, and indeed for the alleviation of their concern about other problems.

The other medical conditions that are more likely to occur at older ages, such as hypertension, heart disease, chronic bronchitis, renal disease, fibroids and joint diseases, may complicate the pregnancy.

Complications of Pregnancy and Delivery

As Fig. 3 shows, maternal mortality increases with age (Department of Health and Social Security, 1975). Whereas maternal mortality in

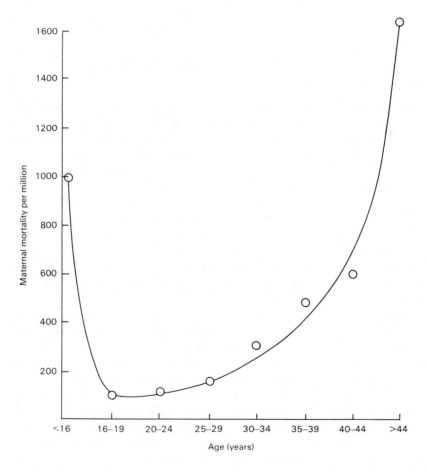

FIG. 3. Maternal mortality per million plotted against maternal age in years.

general has fallen considerably during the last 50 years, the reduction has been mainly among younger women, as Berry's (1977) study of American data demonstrates (Table I). In particular, the risk of dying

Table I
Ratios of the minimum age-specific rate of maternal mortality to each age-specific rate in the years 1917, 1927, 1937, 1947, 1957, and 1967.

Year	Age						
	15−19	20−24	25−29	30−34	35−39	40−44	45−49
1917	1·5	1·0	1·1	1·4	1·9	2·4	2·9
1927	1·4	1·0	1·2	1·5	2·2	2·9	4·1
1937	1·4	1·0	1·2	1·8	2·6	3·4	5·2
1947	1·4	1·0	1·3	2·0	3·4	5·8	10·8
1957	1·5	1·0	1·6	3·1	5·2	7·9	19·2
1967	1·3	1·0	1·3	2·7	4·5	8·2	19·5

from complications of toxaemia, haemorrhage, pulmonary embolism and cardiac disease increases greatly with maternal age (Department of

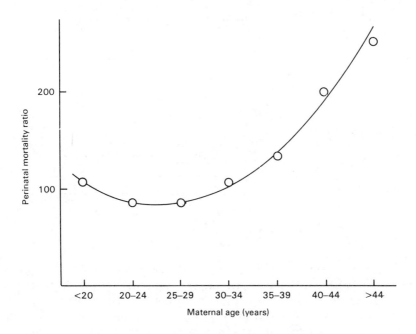

FIG. 4. Perinatal mortality ratio plotted against maternal age in years.

Health and Social Security, 1975). Not only is the risk of mortality increased for the mother, but so is the risk for the child (Chamberlain, 1975), for perinatal mortality also increases with age of mother (Fig. 4). There may also be an increase in risk of foetal loss after 20 weeks with increasing maternal age, independent of parity (Selvin and Garfinkel, 1976).

As regards morbidity, Fig. 5 shows the increase in essential hypertension with age. The apparent drop in women aged 40 and more was due to the small numbers in this age group. It will be noted that pre-eclampsia did not increase with age as markedly as hypertension (Chamberlain, 1978). For the elderly primiparous woman, or for those who have had a gap of more than ten years since their last pregnancy, placental insufficiency is more common and the incidence of prematurity is doubled (Morrison, 1975; Kajanoja and Widholm, 1978).

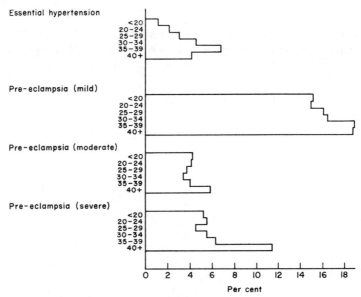

FIG. 5. Hypertension related to age.

For these reasons the older woman will need more care during her pregnancy. She will have to attend the antenatal clinic regularly at shorter intervals, and will need more rest than her younger counterpart. It is helpful to confirm gestational age and to monitor foetal growth with ultrasound, and if necessary with such placental function tests as may be required.

Similarly, more care will be required during the labour itself, and the foetus must be monitored. The incidence of Caesarean section is much increased (Soumplis and Lolis, 1969; Morrison, 1975; Kajanoja and Widholm 1978).

Foetal Abnormality

It is now established that the incidence of trisomy 21 increases with maternal age (Fig. 6) (Erickson, 1978). There is also an increase in some sex chromosome aneuploidies (Carothers et al., 1978). In addition, the incidence of neural tube defects also increases with age (Janerich, 1973).

The total malformation rate shows no consistent relationship with paternal age independent of maternal age. There are, however, some higher rates of malformation at the extreme of the range of paternal ages (50 and over) but the numbers are small, for example oral clefts, polydactyly, syndactyly, achondroplasia, arachnodactyly, Apert's syndrome, and possibly low birth weight (Polednak, 1976). Many of these conditions are thought to be monogenic, and this increased

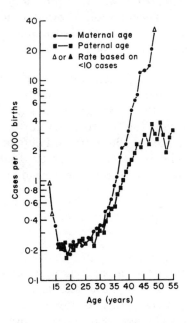

FIG. 6. Down syndrome rates against parental age, NIS surveillance area 1961–1966.

incidence with paternal age to reflect an increase in mutation rate (Roberts, 1979).

After Delivery and Subsequent Development of the Offspring

The older mother may become more tired more easily, and have more anxieties over her child, especially if it is her first. Both she and her husband will find it more difficult to adapt to parenthood. As the child grows older it may suffer from isolation due to the fact that its parents do not have many friends with children of the same age. This is less of a problem when the child goes to school, but even there the child may feel somewhat different from others whose parents participate more enthusiastically in physical activities. There is of course an increased risk of parental death, which can have a profound effect on the child.

It is very difficult to separate out the effect of parental age alone on the child's development. The parents tend to be more intelligent, of a higher social class, have better housing and smaller families, which all tend to produce a more intelligent child. In Amsterdam, a survey of male 19-year-old recruits from two-child families, controlled for social class according to father's occupation, showed a significant association between higher intelligence and increased maternal age, which could not be related to socio-economic or regional variations (Zybert *et al.*, 1978).

Many smaller and less well-controlled retrospective studies have shown slight increases in a number of conditions, such as dyslexia (Jayasekara and Street, 1978), schizophrenia (Dalen, 1977), homosexuality (Abe and Moran, 1969), neuroses (Norton, 1952), personality problems (Rowley and Stone, 1966), mental deficiency (Lilienfeld and Pasamanick, 1956) and epilepsy (Hertoft *et al.*, 1958). The evidence in these and other similar reports should be viewed critically.

Conclusion

The older parent will need more attention and help during her pregnancy and delivery. The prenatal diagnosis of chromosome abnormality and neural tube defects must be offered. She is more likely to have an operative delivery than her younger counterpart. However, with good care, one can expect a favourable outcome and, in the absence of associated diseases, an older woman need not be deterred from having a pregnancy later in life provided that she will accept the necessary investigations and greater supervision.

References

Abe, K. and Moran, P.A.P. (1969). Parental age of homosexuals. *British Journal of Psychiatry*, 115, 313–317.

Berry, L.G. (1977). Age and parity influences on maternal mortality: United States 1919–1969. *Demography*, 14. 297–310.

Carothers, A.D., Collyer, S., De Mey, R. and Frackiewicz, A. (1978). Parental age and birth order in the aetiology of some sex chromosome aneuploidies. *Annals of Human Genetics*, 41, 277–287.

Cartwright, A. (1976). *How Many Children?* London: Routledge & Kegan Paul.

Chamberlain, R. (1975). *British Births 1970*, Vol. 1. *The First Week of Life*. London: Heinemann Medical Books.

Chamberlain, R. (1978). *British Births 1970*, Vol. 2. *Obstetric Care*. London: Heinemann Medical Books.

Dalen, P. (1977). Maternal age and incidence of schizophrenia in the Republic of Ireland. *British Journal of Psychiatry*, 131, 301–305.

Department of Health and Social Security (1975). *Report on Confidential Enquiries into Maternal Deaths in England and Wales 1970–1972*. Health and Social Subjects 11. London: H.M.S.O.

Erickson, J.D. (1978). Down syndrome, paternal age, maternal age and birth order. *Annals of Human Genetics*, 41, 289–298.

Hertoft, P., Leine, L. and Semonsen, H. (1958). Aetiological factors in cryptogenic epilepsy. *Acta Psychiatrica Neurologica Scandinavia*, 33, 296–299.

Janerich, D.T. (1973). Maternal age and spina bifida: longitudinal versus cross-sectional analysis. *American Journal of Epidemiology*, 96, 389–395.

Jayasekara, R. and Street, J. (1978). Parental age and parity in dyslexic boys. *Journal of Biosocial Science*, 10, 255–261.

Kajanoja, P. and Widholm, O. (1978). Pregnancy and delivery in women aged forty and over. *Obstetrics and Gynaecology*, 51, 47–51.

Lilienfeld, A.M. and Pasamanick, B. (1956). The association of maternal and fetal factors with the development of mental deficiency. II. Relationships of maternal age, birth order, previous reproductive loss and degree of mental deficiency. *American Journal of Mental Deficiency*, 60, 557–568.

Morrison, I. (1975). The elderly primigravida. *American Journal of Obstetrics and Gynecology*, 121, 465–470.

Norton, A. (1952). Incidence of neuroses related to maternal age and birth order. *British Journal of Social Medicine*, 6, 253–255.

Office of Population Censuses and Surveys (1978a). *Birth Statistics, England and Wales 1976*. Series FMI, No. 3. London: HMSO.

Office of Population Censuses and Surveys (1978b). *Legal Abortion in England and Wales*. London: HMSO.

Polednak, A.P. (1976). Paternal age in relation to selected birth defects. *Human Biology*, 48, 727–739.

Roberts, D.F. (1979). Genetics and aging in man. In *Fertility in Middle Age,* edited by A.S. Parkes, M.A. Herbertson and J. Cole, pp. 177–195. *Journal of Biosocial Science,* Supplement No. 6. Cambridge: The Galton Foundation.

Rowley, V.N. and Stone, F.B. (1966). Children's behavioural problems and mother's age. *Journal of Psychology,* **63**, 229–235.

Selvin, S. and Garfinkle, J. (1976). Paternal age, maternal age and birth order and the risk of a fetal loss. *Human Biology,* **48**, 223–230.

Soumplis, A.C. and Lolis, D.E. (1969). Elderly primipara. *International Surgery,* **52**, 340–344.

Zybert, P., Stein, Z. and Belmont, L. (1978). Maternal age and children's ability. *Perceptual and Motor Skills,* **47**, 815–818.

Subject Index